The only scientific book of its kind on juices for those who desire to maintain health, preserve youthfulness, rejuvenate their bodies and get relief from diseases

GALA

JUICE-DIET FOR PERFECT HEALTH

By

Dr. Dhiren Gala

B.Sc., D.H.M.S., D.O., D.Ac.,
C.G.O., C.C.H., A.R.S.H.

**Recipient of a gold medal for extraordinary
work in the field of Alternative Therapeutics**

With

Dr. D. R. Gala
N.D., D.N.O., D.C.O.

Dr. Sanjay Gala
M.B. (BOM.), M.S. (ENT)

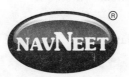

Knowledge is wealth

NAVNEET PUBLICATIONS (INDIA) LIMITED

Navneet House	**Navneet Bhavan**
Gurukul Road, Memnagar,	Bhavanishankar Road,
Ahmadabad – 380 052.	Dadar, Mumbai – 400 028.
Phone : 6630 5000	Phone : 6662 6565

DHANLAL BROTHERS DISTRIBUTORS

70, Princess Street, Mumbai – 400 002.
Phone : 2201 7027 / 2205 3716

G 4507

Visit us at : www.navneet.com | e-mail : npil@navneet.com | **Price : Rs. 65.00**

Dr. D. R. Gala

1st Floor, Abbas Bldg. 'A',
Near Tilak Market, Jalbhai Lane,
Harkishandas Hospital Road,
Grant Road (East), Mumbai – 400 004.
Phone : 2386 7275
Time : 4.00 to 7.00 p.m.

[6 – 2 – 2010 (19) : 7]

PREFACE

All of us wish to live a healthy and happy life free from all diseases, but very few of us make right and really serious efforts in this direction. It is a pity that man, the most intelligent and clever of all living beings, is unable to check the deterioration of his health. This is because the life of modern man is far removed from nature. We do not realise that healthy life is possible only by following the rules of nature. Life is nature's gift to us and we can make the most of this gift only by reverting to Mother Nature.

Nature has provided a variety of food items to us, but instead of including them in their natural form in our diet, we go for hot and spicy food prepared as per various recipes given out by modern books on cookery, little realising that they cater to our tastes rather than to our dietary needs.

No wonder then we have to go for more and more medicines and drugs to save ourselves from the harmful effects of such unnatural foods. It is really deplorable that not only the common man but also the men of medicine and dietetics have remained indifferent to food on which our whole existence, life and well-being depend. It is high time we pay proper attention to our food and cultivate proper food habits to prevent ill-health, since prevention is better than cure.

It has been found that the diet of raw food and juice can help us remain healthy. Juice-diet, especially, can cure us of chronic diseases and keep our mind and body healthy. It is heartening to note that of late our awareness of the importance of juices in our diet has been increasing and that having realized the food value of juices, more and more people are taking juices in their diet.

The results of experiments and research carried on in western countries in the subject of juice-diet are most gratifying and are sure to bring a ray of hope for the health of mankind.

It has been our endeavour to provide in this book information on Juice-diet based on scientific experiments. We are confident that the book will serve as a practical and useful guide to those who desire to prevent diseases and improve their health with the help of juice-diet.

–Authors

CONTENTS

PART 1
Page No.

1. Introduction ... 5
2. Food – Cooked and Uncooked ... 11
3. Raw Juice Therapy ... 29
4. How to Obtain all the Nutrients from Juices ... 37
5. Juice-Fasting ... 44
6. Ten Important Commandments for Juice-diet ... 50

PART 2

Contents and Qualities of Fruits and Vegetables

1. Apple ... 54
2. Beetroot ... 56
3. Bel *(Bilifal)* ... 58
4. Bitter Gourd *(Karela)* ... 59
5. Cabbage ... 61
6. Carrot ... 64
7. Coconut ... 70
8. Cucumber ... 72
9. Emblica Myrobalan *(Amla)* ... 74
10. Fig ... 76
11. French Beans ... 78
12. Garlic ... 79
13. Ginger ... 82
14. Grapes ... 84
15. Guava ... 89
16. Jambul ... 91
17. Lemon ... 92
18. Melon ... 95
19. Onions ... 97
20. Orange ... 99
21. Papaya ... 102
22. Pineapple ... 105
23. Pomegranate ... 107
24. Potatoes ... 108
25. Pumpkin ... 111
26. Sweet Lemon ... 112
27. Tomatoes ... 113
28. Turmeric ... 115
29. Watermelon ... 117
30. White Gourd *(Dudhi)* 118
31. Green Leafy Vegetables ... 120
32. The Wheatgrass juice ... 130
33. Honey ... 141
34. Rejuvenation by Milk 144
35. Rejuvenation by Thick Buttermilk ... 151

PART 3

1. Juice-treatment in Different Diseases ... 155
2. Blends of Juices for Pleasure ... 165
3. Some Cases Showing Successful Experimentation of Juice-diet ... 167
4. Epilogue ... 172
   * Index ... 174

PART 1

1. INTRODUCTION

Every therapy, that has no faith in the efficacy of medicine, has conceded the importance of food for a healthy life. Some of the eminent experts of modern medicine now lay emphasis on food-therapy. It has been invariably established that the use of improper food is perhaps the root cause of every disease. Raw food, vegetables and fruits are better for health than cooked or fried food or food prepared in any other way. Compared to milk, juices of grapes, carrots, strawberries and raspberries are more effective for health and nourishment. Vegetable and fruit juices help to cure such diseases as cannot be cured by modern medicine and various therapies.

Nevertheless, it cannot be denied that there are yet many doctors and patients who show their reluctance to the above facts.

Naturopathy or Nature-cure has been gaining increasing popularity during the last few years, and particularly, juice-therapy has established its exclusive importance in Nature-cure. Juice-therapy has no alternative for alleviating common illness as well as chronic or hard-to-cure diseases. Not only does it enable you to enjoy a healthy life but also it helps you to rejuvenate yourself. Juice-diet and raw food have proved considerably effective to the cases where other modern therapies have failed. Poisonous drugs like thalidomide, after their prolonged use for many years, have now been discarded. These harmful drugs are now being replaced by non-medicinal treatment like Nature-cure, and more and more doctors and patients are inclined towards the acceptance of the use of nourishing food, vegetables and fruit-juices for the maintenance of health and cure of diseases.

Man born in the lap of Nature has now recognized the right direction of cultivating the delight of the body and the mind and of maintaining health by using natural food and juices. Mankind will find the source of real hope and joy in this new trend.

It is now imperative for all to choose juice-diet or juice-therapy in place of modern medicines because toxic elements contained in these medicines are harmful to the diseased and very often they prolong illness instead of curing it.

Improper food and habits – fatal to health : We all desire happiness, peace and prosperity but the basic condition of achieving them is good health. How many of us observe the basic rules of physical and mental health and take proper food and follow good habits?

We Indians are fatalists. Therefore, we live a life, leaving to God, Almighty solely to take care of our health and well-being. We don't think of the right food and eat. Consequently, when we fall ill, we are used to finding fault with fate. Our motto of life is 'the soul is immortal and the body is transient'. Such beliefs have made us careless towards our health. We rarely observe the basic principles of sound health. A negligible illness, and we rush to a doctor and administer poisonous drugs into our body. May be, these poisonous drugs give immediate relief, but this relief is short-lived. When the same ailment recurs, we are compelled to take stronger drugs in large doses with the result that several new diseases spring up out of one and we are entrapped in such a vicious circle that it is hard to get out of it.

But do not despair; there is one simple but effective way to get rid of the vicious circle of medicines. At the outset, we must clearly understand the fact that the origin of man's major or minor illnesses is his improper dietic habits. We maintain physical and mental fitness through the consumption of proper and wholesome food. Raw food is the main force of preserving our health. According to Dr. Robert Mckarison, an eminent physician, a proper diet is the best of all the medicines produced in the world. In the same way we can say that an improper diet is the cause of a disease.

If we accept these two facts, our health is in our hands. Our present diet is based on taste. If we change it, we can save thousands of rupees which are otherwise spent on medicines. The best diet is that which maintains our health in a natural way, nourishes the limbs and the organs of the body, makes them active and supplies whatever is deficient in the body.

Whether a particular diet is proper or improper should be considered carefully. It is advisable to go for raw food in comparison to cooked food for the betterment of health. Compared to fried and boiled vegetables, unprocessed vegetables and their juices give much more nutrition and vitality. Sunripened fruits and raw food are considered more beneficial to health than canned fruits and juices, biscuits, bread, pickles, sweets, etc. because minerals and enzymes can be obtained only from fresh vegetables, fruits and natural food and they are essential for nourishment and health. Cooking destroys vitamins, enzymes and minerals contained in food-grains, vegetables and fruits. Sugar, salt and other delicious condiments, when added, make the food indigestible and without nutrients. Besides, diets with improper combinations such as fruit salad, rice-pudding with pulses, milk with onions and garlic impair our health.

The number and varieties of items of eatables and drinks are multiplying day by day. Moreover, we become gluttonous at late night parties. Today's life is a life of haste, hurry, bustle and mental tension. Under this stress we are now used to taking refreshments every now and then throughout the day. Consequently the mode of man's life has become irregular and discordant. Biological rhythm of the body is endangered by irregular timings of eating, drinking, sleeping and walking. These irregularities disarrange the excretory functioning of the body. This is the reason why constipation, insomnia, bodyache and headache are the common complaints of today. The use of intoxicating substances like tea, coffee, tobacco, bhang, ganja (hemp), etc. is also the cause of the accumulation of toxins and other harmful elements in the body. The system of adding colour, taste and flavour to food and the various processes through which it passes destroy its life-giving nutrients. And look at the manufacturers; after food is processed, synthetic vitamins are added to make it nutritious. But all these additives and processed foods are injurious to health.

The diet consisting of raw or boiled food, raw vegetables, fruits and fresh fruit-juices is proper and desirable for health. Among all diets juice-diet is considered best for health and vitality.

Sugar – a sweet poison : Modern therapeutics recommend restriction on the consumption of sugar for the purpose of maintaining health. The Ayurveda and the naturopathy recommend avoidance of sugar from diet. Harmless substances like honey and fruits should be substituted for sugar. Jaggery is produced from sugar-cane-juice. White sugar is also produced from sugar-cane-juice through modern process. Considering their nutritious elements, sugar-cane-juice is more beneficial to health than jaggery, but white sugar has no role as a nutrient.

One of the causes of good health of our ancestors was the absence of white sugar in their diet. They maintained the health and energy because they obtained as much fructose as they wanted from raw food, vegetables and fruits. Professor John Yudkin of England has minutely studied the effects of sugar in human body. He states that there is no physiological requirement for sugar. The calories and energy required for the body are easily available from fruits, vegetables and grains.

The constitution of our blood is alkaline. So dieticians advise us to eat edibles containing minerals. Sugar and sweets, after digestion leave acidic residue in the body which is harmful and injurious to health. The chemical process made upon sugar for whitening and purifying it destroys its nutritious properties. There is little or no amount of vitamins and minerals in sugar.

The consumption of huge amount of white sugar has led to diseases like dental decay and caries, diabetes, cardiac trouble and hypoglycemia (low blood sugar). The reckless use of sugar leads to migraine, dermatitis and renal disorders. Moreover, sugar increases the amount of cholesterol in the blood. Cholesterol accumulates in the inner surface of the arteries which consequently become narrow and hard. The heart has to work vigorously to push blood into such narrow arteries. Consequently the heart becomes exhausted and weak. Sometimes it fails.

Thus, the excessive use of sugar has adverse effects on health. Not only that, it also interrupts the smooth functioning of the body and the mind and leads to various diseases. That is why sugar is considered a sweet poison by dieticians.

Salt – a redundant constituent of food : If sugar is considered a sweet poison, salt is considered a mineral poison. The intake of salt with food causes untoward effects in the body and to eliminate it the kidneys have to labour. If the excessive intake of salt continues, the kidneys become weak and damaged and sometimes they fail in their work.

It is true that salt is an essential constituent for taste. But excessive consumption of salt proves to be detrimental to health. Because of the popular belief that food cannot be cooked without salt, there is hardly an item in our diet which is saltless. In fact, according to one expert dietician, salt is not at all necessary for either life or health. In other words, there is no physiological need for salt.

More and more dieticians and physicians have now begun to concede that salt is one of the causes of diseases which man suffers from. Excess salt, it is claimed, causes improper calcium absorption. Dr. James Braithwaite claims that salt does harm because it is not a food but an inorganic chemical which improperly stimulates cell metabolism.

Here is a list of various conditions or illnesses said to be caused by salt : headache, insomnia, migraine, heart disease, hives, kidney ailments, dropsy, cirrhosis of the liver, cold, sinus conditions, hearing problems, epilepsy, rheumatism and obesity. Many medical experts and other authorities have pointed to salt as a factor in the causation of cancer. Dr. Frederick Marwood investigated over 100 cancer patients and in every instance, excepting one, he found the victims had been abnormally fond of salt and salted foods.

The human body requires two grains of salt per day and that can be obtained from only 50 grams of vegetables. A diet containing vegetables and fruits supplies sufficient natural salt to the body and no additional salt is required.

Salt has more disadvantages than advantages. A labourer, however, might need additional salt to replace the salts lost in perspiration. If he takes no additional salt, he may suffer from bodyache, muscular cramps and exhaustion.

A complete omission of salt from the diet has been found to cure insomnia and bring sound sleep. Persons suffering from high blood pressure are benefited when they minimise the intake of salt. If we minimise the use of salt in our daily diet, our health will be improved. On the other hand, excess use of salt will create a lot of diseases and complications in our body.

JUICE-DIET FOR PERFECT HEALTH

2. FOOD – COOKED AND UNCOOKED

Eating cooked food is a very old tradition. This tradition of cooking food formed by our ancestors thousands of years ago is being continued by us today. No creature on the earth except man cooks its food. This may be the reason why creatures other than man do not become the victims of illness.

Food when cooked loses its life-giving nutrients and becomes lifeless. There is no possibility of getting energy, health or nourishment from this lifeless food. Life begets life. Food without life cannot bestow life. On the contrary, it makes the existing living lifeless.

According to Dr. George J. Druce of Chicago, cooked food is mankind's oldest addiction. Most of the physical and mental ailments are due to the consumption of cooked food.

The popular belief that food is required only for providing calories and energy to the body and keeping it active is firmly and deeply rooted. But those who believe in this are unaware of the fact that the body continuously suffers wear and tear. Old tissue-cells are being destroyed and to replace them new tissue-cells are being generated. This process of reconstruction is necessary for life and it depends upon the nutritious quality of food which we consume. Our food must contain vitamins, minerals and enzymes to keep the reconstruction work going on. Moreover, protein, carbohydrates and fats contained in food require vitamins and enzymes for their assimilation. In the process of heating food, vitamins and enzymes contained in food are lost to a great extent.

Food taken solely on the basis of taste cannot fulfil the requirements of the body. It is true that cooked food becomes soft and also delicious because of condiments, sweetening, etc. We are prone to eating such food more than required. This overeating causes indigestion followed by other diseases

Cooked food not only loses its vitamins and enzymes but also it undergoes many untoward changes. The protein and the carbohydrates in cooked food are not easily digestible. They are not easily absorbed in the intestines. Thus, cooked food becomes deficient in nutrients. It may perhaps give some nourishment to healthy persons, but for the old and the sick it is useless.

Can we not minimize our love for cooked food and select raw or natural food in its place? Many persons fear that raw food causes heaviness, pain and gas in the abdomen, but their fear is baseless. It has been proved through experiments that raw food is digested within three or four hours, whereas cooked food takes five to six hours for digestion. But fruit and vegetable juices are digested within 25 to 30 minutes and are quickly assimilated into blood.

The above facts prove that raw food and live juices are most suited to the body and they stimulate the process of reconstruction. Precious nutrients are destroyed when food is cooked. But if grains are sprouted, there is a considerable increase in their nutrients. In sprouted cereals there is a 600% increase in vitamins like thiamine, pentothinic acid, niacine etc. We get vitamins 'A' and 'C' from sprouted cereals. Sprouted grains and pulses are very useful for the speedy growth of a child and for increasing a nursing mother's milk.

It is an indisputable fact that if we do away with traditional culture of cooked food and accept raw food as even half the quantity of our diet, our health will go on improving day by day.

Essential elements for health : Even though the subject-matter of the book is juice diet, it will not be out of place to discuss certain essential ingredient of diet. Food should be consumed for keeping the body active and healthy. Man can select proper diet only when he knows what constituents of food are necessary for the body. One should eat only that food, the constituents of which are congenial to one. These constituents should rejuvenate the body besides maintaining health. Diseases are caused because of deficiencies of certain essential constituents. If this is known to us, we shall never eat dispensable food. This kind of understanding of and viewpoint on the system and substance of diet should be cultivated.

With a view to making one's life happy with healthy and active body one's daily diet should normally consist of the following constituents :

(1) **Carbohydrates** : The most important function of the carbohydrates is to provide fuel and energy to the body. The carbohydrates include sugar and starch. This constituent of food is available from all kinds of food-grains (cereals). Flour devoid of husk, polished rice, white sugar, etc., retain their carbohydrates but lose most of the vitamins and minerals. They also do not contain roughage. Processed carbohydrates and the carbohydrates taken in excess reduce the power of digestion and place unnecessary pressure on other organs of the body. Hence we should try to reduce from our diet the quantum of processed food except few substances containing natural carbohydrates.

(2) **Fat** : Fat provides heat to the body. Compared with animal fats (milk, ghee, meat) vegetable fats (oil-seeds, edible oils) are better digested and are comparatively harmless. Animal fats have saturated fatty acids and lead to accumulation of cholesterol in the arteries with the result that the latter become hard and narrow. This invites diseases like high blood pressure, heart disease, etc. It is, therefore, advisable to take food with less fats and that, also prepared in vegetable oils containing unsaturated fats.

(3) **Protein** : Proteins should be given an important place in our diet as they are necessary for the growth, development and reconstruction of the body. Twenty-two types of amino acids constitute proteins. Some of amino acids are produced in the body. The rest should be obtained from food.

A proper combination of various pulses gives us excellent proteins required for the body.

(4) The importance of vitamins : The word vitamin is derived from 'vital' which means indispensable for life. This fact throws light on the value of vitamins. Until the beginning of this century nobody knew anything about vitamins. Physiologists, that time, thought that men could live on a diet consisting of proteins, carbohydrates, fats and minerals in required quantities and that the body required no other nutrients. Then experiments were performed on mice. They were kept on pure proteins, carbohydrates, fats and minerals. In a few days it was found that they had stopped growing. Gradually their body began to wear out and in the end they died. This experiment established that in addition to the constituents mentioned above, some other elements were required for life. Afterwards when these elements were discovered, they were called vitamins. Vitamins 'A', 'B', 'C', 'D', 'E', 'K' and 'P' have been discovered so far.

Vitamins are organic chemical substances required in minute quantity for the process of metabolism in the body. The body itself cannot produce these substances. A brief description of the vitamins is given below.

Vitamin 'A'–Retinol (Antixerophthalmia vitamin; growth vitamin) : Vitamin 'A' in its complete and pure form can be obtained only from animals. However, its provitamin, known as carotene, is available in large quantity from vegetables. Vitamin 'A' is useful to the body in various ways : (1) It is necessary for the process of metabolism occurring in every cell of the body. (2) It is necessary for the growth of the body. When the quantity of vitamin 'A' in the diet of mice was increased, it was noticed that life-span of mice increased[1]. (3) It is essential for eye-sight. Deficiency of vitamin 'A' causes night-blindness. (4) The most serious symptoms due to its lack are a drying up of the skin, teeth troubles, the burning

1. Henry C. Sherman, Ph. D.–The Nutritional Importance of Life, p. 184, Columbia

of mucous membrane, the loss of weight and kidney stones appearing in the urinary tract. (5) The vitamin 'A' deficiency causes diseases like swelling of the body, excessive increase of uric acid in blood, anemia, development of respiratory infections and infections of the ears and nose.

Green leafy vegetables, cabbage, red and yellow fruits and vegetables contain vitamin 'A' in sufficient quantity. This vitamin is fat-soluble. So it cannot be assimilated completely if the food lacks in fat. Of course, the body has a reserved quantity of fat which assists the assimilation of vitamin 'A'. Vitamin 'A' is stable to heat but if exposed to continuous high temperatures over 100 degrees centigrade, it is destroyed.

Vitamin 'D' : Some substances have a quality to prevent rickets, a disease of children. These substances which resemble the secretions of adrenal cortex are called sterols. Some of these substances, when come into contact with ultra-violet rays, turn into vitamin 'D'.

7-dehydro cholesterol lying in the human skin is converted into vitamin 'D' when come into contact with the sun-rays. Thus the human body itself is able to produce vitamin 'D'. It is found in milk. It is fat-soluble. It is not affected by moderate heat or oxygen in the atmosphere.

Vitamin 'D' is essential for the health of bones and the teeth. It is needed for the proper utilization of calcium and phosphorus. The deficiency of vitamin 'D' causes rickets in children. In this disease, the bones become soft, the spinal column and the bones of the arms and legs bend and the teeth suffer from caries. This ailment in persons of advanced age is called 'osteomalasia'.

Vitamin 'K' : By conversion to prothrombin in the liver this vitamin maintains the normal rate of blood coagulation by regulating the prothrombin level. Vitamin 'K' is also fat-soluble. It is sparingly soluble in water.

Vitamin 'K' is found in green and fresh leafy vegetables. Moreover, it is manufactured in the intestines by the bacterial flora that inhabits this organ. The deficiency of vitamin 'K' causes poor clotting of blood and hemorrhagic tendencies.

Vitamin 'C' (Ascorbic acid) : Ascorbic acid is one kind of sugar which is very much useful for the body. It bestows youthfulness and efficiency in work. It is essential for the health of the teeth, the bones and the gums. It strengthens the arteries, prevents hemorrhage and promotes healing of wounds. It is necessary for blood metabolism and thus useful in anemia. Dr. Reisser, an eminent orthopaedic surgeon of Possadena, states that the food which contains vitamin 'C' can prevent the attack of poliomyelitis. It increases the resistance of the body to disease.

This vitamin is considerably destroyed by heat. It is water-soluble. Hence the water used for cooking vegetables should not be discarded. The human body itself cannot produce this vitamin.

The deficiency of vitamin 'C' in the body causes a disease called scurvy. Moreover, this deficiency also causes tooth-decay, gum-troubles, rarifaction of bones, loss of weight and infertility.

This vitamin is found in citrus and sweet fruits and green leafy vegetables. Though potatoes contain a small amount of vitamin 'C', their large consumption supplies sufficient vitamin 'C'.

Vitamin 'B' : The vitamin 'B' complex is composed of many constituents. They include thiamine, niacin, riboflavin, pyrtidoxine, folate and B_{12}. There is another complex containing constituents such as choline, pantothenic acid, biotine, inositol, p-aminobenzoic acid (PABA), panguamic acid and amygdalin (laetrile). The function of these latter constituents remains still unknown.

Vitamin 'B' complex is water-soluble and very useful to the body.

Vitamin 'B$_1$' (Thiamine) : This vitamin stimulates appetite. It activates the muscles and is antineurotic vitamin. It is essential for the metabolism and digestion of food. Experiments show that the deficiency of thiamine increases piruvic acid in the blood which reduces the working capacity and efficiency of the heart. The deficiency of this vitamin causes a disease called beri-beri.

Vitamin 'B$_1$' is found in pulses (cereals), yeast, sprouted wheat, unpolished rice, soyabeans, milk, green leafy vegetables and fruits and vegetables. This vitamin is destroyed when food articles are cooked in open air.[1]

Vitamin 'B$_2$' (Riboflavin) : This vitamin too is necessary for intracellular metabolism. It is necessary for growth, health, development of resistance-power and longevity. It preserves youthfulness and keeps old age away. It strengthens the muscles, increases the eye-sight and contributes to proper digestion. Its water-solubility is moderate. It is destroyed when exposed to light.

Its deficiency deranges the working of the salivary and pituitary glands, and decreases metabolism. The prolonged deficiency of this vitamin causes diseases of the digestive system, weakness of the muscles and skin diseases.

This vitamin can be obtained from milk, yeast, soyabeans, sprouted wheat, papaya, banana, etc.

Niacin (Nicotinic acid and Nicotinamide) : This vitamin is necessary for appetite and mental health. It is found in foodgrains, milk, yeast, potatoes, etc. If bran is removed from the flour of food-grains most of niacin is lost. The body also produces this vitamin in very little quantity. Its deficiency causes a disease called pellagra. Besides, insomnia, headache and skin diseases also result from its deficiency.

---

1. Jesse Feiring wiliams., M. D.– Personal Hygiene Applied, p. 204, Philadelphia

Vitamin 'B$_6$' (Pyridoxine) : It is a combination of three constituents and is believed to be necessary for the metabolism of proteins. It is found in sufficient quantities in milk, vegetables and husk of food-grains. Its deficiency causes ailments of the skin, the liver, the blood-vessels and the nervous system.

Vitamin 'B$_{12}$' : The deficiency of this vitamin adversely affects the production of DNA, a very valuable element of the cells of the body. Its deficiency causes one type of anemia and degenerative changes of the spinal column.

Folate : This vitamin is found in green leafy vegetables. Its deficiency causes anemia and malfunctioning of the digestive system.

The above-mentioned constituent vitamins of vitamin 'B' complex are more effective collectively. They can tolerate moderate heat but are destroyed if exposed to heat for a prolonged time. Soda used in cooking also leads to their destruction.

Vitamin 'E'.: This is an antisterility vitamin. It is claimed that conception cannot occur without an adequate quantity of vitamin 'E'. Its deficiency causes repeated abortions. This vitamin is useful for the metabolism of fats. It is believed that this vitamin controls catabolism. It prevents heart-disease, diabetes, asthma, thrombosis, diseases of the blood-vessels and degenerative changes of the spine.

It will be procured from sprouted wheat, vegetables, dried fruits, etc.

Vitamin 'P' (Bioflavonoids) : This vitamin is necessary for maintaining health of the blood-vessels and for normalising blood pressure.

It is found in citrus fruits and vegetables.

Individual characteristics of various vitamins have been described above. But experiments have confirmed of better results when vitamins are used in combination. The presence of one vitamin increases the efficacy of another vitamin.

Our body itself also is capable of producing some vitamins. There are several benevolent symbiotic bacteria in the intestines, which produce vitamins for the body.[1] These bacteria particularly produce vitamins 'B', 'E' and 'K'. Antibiotic drugs destroy these bacteria and so we should use these drugs cautiously.

The body can store or accumulate vitamins 'A', 'D', 'E' and 'K'. When need arises, these vitamins are available from the body-storage. However, vitamins 'B' and 'C' cannot be stored in the body. So we should be careful to see that we obtain these vitamins from our daily diet.

Of all vitamins, vitamin 'C' is destroyed most rapidly and easily. All the vitamins are destroyed to a greater or lesser degree when exposed to heat or air (oxygen) or if food is stored for a long time. If a banana is cut into pieces or is grated and kept for some time, it loses about 50% of its vitamin 'C'.[2]

Vitamin 'A' is stable to moderate heat but if the food is cooked open, it is destroyed immediately.

As stated above, some vitamins ('B', 'C') are water-soluble and some are fat-soluble. The body can obtain vitamins 'B' and 'C' easily but if the diet is short of fats, the body finds it difficult to get vitamin 'A', 'D' and 'E'.[3] If oil is used as purgative, vitamins 'A' and 'D' are discharged, with stools. So it is not advisable to use oil for purgative purposes.

Countless experiments have proved that vitamins are most effective when taken in their natural forms. 'Journal of Nutrition' has published a report of an experiment conducted by Dr. E. M. Todhunter and Dr. A. S. Fatzer. These two scientists administered natural and synthetic vitamin 'C' to some college-girls. The quantity given was the same every

1. Sir John Conybeare, F. R. C. P. and W. N. Mann, M. D. F. R. C. P., Textbook of Medicine, p. 264, London
2. Jesse Feiring Williams, M. D., Personal Hygiene Applied, p. 206, Philadelphia
3. Franklin Bicknell, M. D. F. R. C. P., The Vitamins in Medicine, p.12

time. Natural vitamin 'C' (Raspberry juice) was absorbed easily, quickly and completely in the body, whereas synthetic vitamin 'C' was absorbed in a small proportion in the body and that also with difficulty. In one issue of a famous British periodical **'Lancet'**, Dr. A. Elmby and Dr. E. Warburg also have confirmed the same fact. They say that the function of synthetic vitamin 'C' as an antiscorbatic agent is not satisfactory. That is why natural vitamins contained in fruit and vegetable juices assume great importance.

The importance of minerals : As per Webster's International Dictionary, a mineral is a solid homogeneous, crystalline chemical element or compound that results from the inorganic processes of nature.

According to Taber's Cyclopaedic Medical Dictionary, a mineral is a solid inorganic element or compound occurring in nature. It is essential for the formation of cells of the body.

Minerals are essential for maintaining optimal health. The significant role of minerals for maintenance of proper health is emphasized in a report made by Dr. Tom Douglas Spies at an Annual Meeting of the American Medical Association. It is as follows :

'All diseases are caused by chemicals, and all diseases can be cured by chemicals. All the chemicals used by the body are taken in through food. If only we knew enough about them, all diseases could be prevented, and could be cured through their proper use.'

As regards the functions of minerals, the following formation has been compiled through experiments :

(1) Minerals are essential constituents of all cells. (2) They form the greater portion of bones, teeth and nails. (3) They are essential components of respiratory pigments, enzymes and enzyme systems. (4) They regulate the permeability of cell membranes and capillaries. (5) They

regulate the excitability of muscular and nervous tissues. (6) They are essential for regulation of osmotic pressure equilibria. (7) They are necessary for maintenance of proper acid-base balance. (8) They are essential constituents of secretions of glands. (9) They play an important role in water metabolism and regulation of blood volume.

The above list shows that minerals play a very important role in the complex processes going on in the body.

One cannot imagine life without minerals. Man can survive with hunger for a longer period than when kept on food without minerals.[1] In an experiment dogs could not survive for more than 25 to 30 days when kept on food short of minerals.[2]

Approximately 20–30 gm of mineral salts are excreted daily from the body through urine. These must be replaced daily through food intake. Fifteen elements of the various minerals are extremely necessary for the body. Other five to six minerals are considered to be essential for creatures, but there are differences in opinions regarding their utility for man. Minerals and their average quantity found in human body are mentioned below :

Mineral Salt	Quantity	
Calcium	1000	gm.
Phosphorus	780	gm.
Potassium	140	gm.
Sulphur	140	gm.
Sodium	100	gm.
Chlorine	95	gm.
Magnesium	19	gm.
Iron	4.2	gm.
Copper	72	gm.

1. R. N. Chopra, M. D., M. R. C. P., A Handbook of Tropical Therapeutics, p. 154, Calcutta
2. Julius, Ferdinand, M. D.– Diet in Health and Diseases, p. 150, Philadelphia

Mineral Salt	Quantity
Iodine	13 gm.
Manganese	12 gm.
Fluorine	2.6 gm.
Zinc	2.3 gm.
Chromium	2.0 gm.
Cobalt	1.5 gm.

From the above list, it is clear that the last seven minerals are present in very small quantity in the body. Out of the fifteen minerals mentioned in the above list, calcium, phosphorus and iron are most important.

Calcium : The bones and the teeth have approximately 99% of the total calcium of the body.[1] Vitamin 'D' is essential for the metabolism and absorption of calcium in the body. Calcium is necessary for the working of enzymes. It supplies energy for the contraction of the muscles. Calcium prevents swelling and bleeding. Due to the deficiency of calcium, the bones become brittle, the blood-circulation slows down and the blood loses its capacity for coagulation. Mental strain and stress interrupt the capacity of the body for absorbing calcium.

After the age of 55, due to some unknown reasons,the bones begin to lose calcium. This causes osteoporosis. For this, Dr. N. R. Urist advises that in old age one should take 1.0 gm. of calcium per kilogram of body-weight, 1000 International Units of vitamin 'D' and 1.0 to 2.0 gms. of protein daily.

Fenugreek, drumstick and other leafy vegetables, beet, fig, grapes, water-melon, milk, dried fruits, millet, sesame seeds, black beans, etc. have abundant amount of calcium.

Phosphorus : Next to calcium phosphorus is considered to be the most important mineral for human beings. The bones and the teeth contain 75% of the total phosphorus of

1. Micheal G. Wohl, M. D., Dietotherapy, p. 147, Philadelphia

the body. The remaining 25% phosphorus lies in the various parts of the body and does the following important functions :

1. Phosphorus is essential for the growth and nourishment of the body.
2. It activates the digestive juices.
3. It helps the process of metabolism of sygar and fats.
4. It is also essential for the functioning of the brain and the nerves.

The deficiency of phosphorus weakens the teeth and the bones and causes a loss in weight. The body requires a minimum of 1.0 gm. of phosphorus daily.

Phosphorus is available from milk, yeast, dried fruits, soyabean, carrot, guava, dates, etc.

Iron : Approximately 70% of the total iron of the body forms a part of haemoglobin in the red corpuscles of the body. The oxidation going in the body depends on these red corpuscles. 20% iron is preserved in the liver. Besides, the muscles have iron in the form of myoglobine. Iron is found in 'serum transferrin' and some enzymes. Iron is necessary for supplying oxygen, through lungs to each cell of the body. It is also necessary for the respiration of the cells. The deficiency of iron causes anemia. Many a time, due to lack of vitamin 'C' and 'E', the red corpuscles are destroyed. In such cases the body requires more iron. The minimum requirement of iron in the body per day is 12.0 mg. but increases many times in case of pregnancy.

Iron is found in plenty in green leafy vegetables (particularly fenugreek and mint), mango, dates, sesame, millet, grams, soyabeans, mung, black beans, pistachio nuts, etc.

Besides calcium, phosphorus and iron, there are other minerals useful to the body. Their brief description is given below :

Potassium : Potassium is necessary for the constitution of

the cells and the muscles. It maintains the elasticity of the
muscles. The daily potassium requirement of the body is
about 4.0 gms. It is found in garlic, radish, pumpkin,
tomatoes, spinach, guava, apple, milk and potatoes.

Sodium : Sodium helps to produce hydrochloric acid in
the stomach. It prevents the accumulation of calcium in the
muscles. The daily sodium requirement of the body is
approximately 2.0 gm. Its deficiency can lead to formation of
stone in kidney. It is found in sufficient quantity in beet, carrot
and French beans.

Iodine : It is a part of the secretion of the thyroid gland.
Through this secretion, iodine helps in the process of metabolism. Its deficiency causes menstrual troubles. The thyroid
gland does not function properly if the body lacks sufficient
iodine. Iodine deficiency causes a disease called
myxoedema. It causes obesity and the body becomes the
victim of other disorders, such as constipation, drowsiness
and cardiac trouble. Scrofula is a main symptom of the
deficiency of iodine. Iodine is found in sufficient amount in
leafy vegetables.

Magnesium : It is essential for the health of the bones
and the teeth. It maintains functioning capacity of the
muscular system. The minimum quantity of magnesium
required daily by the body is 0.6 gm. It is available from
guava, radish, spinach, potatoes, etc.

Chlorine : Chlorine is essential for the production of
hydrochloric acid in the stomach. It purifies blood and
prevents the joints from being stiff. The body needs 15.0 to
20.0 gm of chlorine daily. Carrot, apricot, beet, French beans,
cabbage, tomatoes, banana, dates, legume, etc., contain
chlorine.

Sulphur : Sulphur is a blood-purifying mineral. It
activates the liver and brightens the skin. 0.3 gm of sulphur is

the daily requirement of the body. It is available from garlic, beet, radish, onion, etc.

Manganese : Manganese subsists particularly in the pancreas, the liver and the hair. It strengthens the muscles and increases the resistance power of the body against disease. It can be procured from garlic, beet, cabbage and guava.

Fluorine : It is essential for the constitution of the bones and the teeth.

Copper : It is necessary for the absorption of iron in the body.

Zinc : It is essential for the health of the prostate gland.

Cobalt : It helps the production of haemoglobin.

Spinach, fenugreek and other leafy vegetables, guava, carrot, beet, potatoes etc., contain all these minerals.

The necessity of enzymes : According to Dr. James B. Sumner, professor of bio-chemistry at the Cornell University, three substances are very vital for perfect health – vitamins, minerals and enzymes. The importance of vitamins and minerals has already been discussed. Now let us consider the importance of enzymes.

An enzyme is a catalyst. It is produced in the live cells. It works as a catalyst even in a very small amount. It means that it aids chemical changes in the body. Every process in the body depends on enzymes. One or more enzymes are necessary for each separate process occurring in the body. Each enzyme has a fixed field of action. Digestion and assimilation– the two important processes of the body– cannot satisfactorily go through without enzymes.

Our body is unable to produce vitamins and minerals, but can produce enzymes. Every animal or vegetable cell can produce enzymes. Enzymes have not been seen yet; but their existence can be realized. It is believed that enzymes are one kind of proteins.

There are many kinds of enzymes. Life without enzymes is not possible. Enzymes help in digestion of food. They decompose food into its different constituents so that they can be assimilated into the body through the intestinal membranes. It is believed that enzymes reconstruct the cells, the glands and the muscles of the body through the digested food. They play a major role in the accumulation of glycogen in the liver and muscles. They help in discharging carbon dioxide from the lungs.

Some particular enzymes help to collect phosphorus in the bones. Certain enzymes produce iron compound in the red corpuscles, others help in the process of blood-coagulation when bleeding takes place. There are certain such enzymes which would attack on the toxins and other unwanted substances in the body. They convert them into urea or uric acid and finally remove them from the body.

Some enzymes can convert proteins into sugar or fats and others can convert fats into carbohydrates. In fact, all the functions of enzymes are not yet fully known.

All natural edible substances possess enzymes. Heat destroys enzymes. Despite this we eat only cooked food, and because of this we are deprived of enzymes. This is one of the reasons why we do not enjoy a long life.

Our body can produce enzymes to its requirement but for that its productive organs have to work hard. In youth this work is accomplished without much difficulty but as we advance in age, the capacity of the organs for doing work is diminished, the production of enzymes cannot cope up with the demand and consequently we become the victims of diseases.

Where is the necessity to tax different organs, when sufficient enzymes for the metabolism in the body are easily available from raw food? Why should we not leave the work of reconstruction of the body to the enzymes contained in raw food? This is the very purpose of nature.

Scientific experiments have proved that the body cannot function properly without enzymes. When the body is not supplied with required quantity of enzymes, it begins to degenerate. Most of dieticians are of the opinion that without enzymes man becomes prematurely old. The research-scholars at the famous Michael Reidge Hospital of Chicago have stated that the saliva of old persons contains only the thirtieth part of enzymes contained in the saliva of young persons.

Dr. Ekart analysed 1200 people's urine samples. He is of the opinion that old peoples' urine contains half of the enzymes in comparison to adults'.

Doctor Berg of Illinois University has proved that when insects become old, they too become deficient in enzymes. Researches conducted by Dr. Sekla and Dr. Folk of Charles University of Prague on bees and mice respectively have established that with the passage of time after youth, the amount of enzymes in the body decreases gradually.

In old age the body cannot produce the required enzymes in sufficient quantities. Hence there is no other alternative except to replenish them from raw live food. It does not mean that children and young persons do not need raw food. The intake of raw food saves the enzyme-producing organs from unnecessary burden and they (organs) remain active throughout the life.

In the digestive system of the human body, enzymes begin to function right from the mouth. The saliva secreted with the process of chewing food contains some enzymes. These enzymes begin the work of digestion. If saliva and digestive juices of the stomach do not contain sufficient enzymes, food causes heaviness in the stomach. The fermentation of food causes gas and uneasiness.

Recently, an enzyme called insulin has become well-known. It is essential for the metabolism of carbohydrates. Its deficiency causes diabetes. Sugar in the body of a diabetic does not get oxidised properly. Hence sugar is found in blood and the urine of a diabetic. The latest researches have pointed out a possibility that the total quantity of insulin in pancreas is limited. If this quantity is exhausted or made exhausted by improper food habits, diabetes is caused.

The following points are worth remembering as the summary of this chapter :

(1) Enzymes are very vital for the body and health. (2) Heat destroys enzymes. (3) The body's own accumulated stock of enzymes is like a bank-balance. If you spend it more than necessary it will sooner be exhausted. A great difficulty arises when enzymes are exhausted. Therefore, to avoid depletion of the limited accumulated stock of enzymes in the body, it is advisable to take natural food and live juices in abundance.

---

3. RAW JUICE THERAPY

Where medicines and injections fail to cure a disease, a proper diet, vegetables and fruit juices show miraculous results. Having been assured of the above fact, Dr. Bircher-Banner, an eminent physician of Switzerland, left his roaring practice and established a nature-cure centre at Zurich. He relieves the people of their ailments by the use of raw food, vegetable and fruit juices.

Raw food, vegetable and fruit-juices should be consumed for general health and well being. But to get relief from a particular disease specific juice therapy should be resorted to under the guidance of an expert.

Dr. Max Gerson has treated cancer-patients with fruit and vegetable juices and saved them from the jaws of death. He states that in the treatment of cancer it is necessary to get the catabolic cells activated. For that, he makes use of plenty of live juices of vegetables.

Fruit-juices are more effective than medicines on the kidney. Juice-therapy is an efficacious cure for the ailments of the liver and the kidney. Cherry-juice bestows marvellous benefits in the cases of gout and arthritis.

A diet containing vegetable and fruit-juices and raw food has been proved a successful experiment for preventing aging and for the rejuvenation of the body. There is no alternative to juice-therapy for the rapid replacement of red corpuscles and cells in the human body.

The treatment given through vegetable and fruit-juices is harmless, reliable and without any side-effects. Even if some-times fruit-juices are taken in abundance, no hyper-vitaminosis can occur. Therefore, it is logical to prefer juice-therapy to any other risk-involving remedy in illness.

Innumerable cells inhabited in the body and billions of blood-corpuscles perish every day. Food is necessary for their replenishment. If the food is natural and combined with vegetable and fruit-juices, this replacement takes place very rapidly. This is most essential in the case of those who are unhealthy and of an advanced age. Elements obtained from raw food and the juices of vegetables and fruits are most essential for maintaining the proper balance of the construction and destruction of the blood-corpuscles and cells. Sugar and other substances contained in them are easily digestible and after their quick absorption in the blood, begin the work of the reconstruction.

Synthetic vitamins and enzymes given to a patient as medicines are not as effective as they are supposed to be, while natural vitamins and enzymes obtained from live juices give wonderful results.

A diet consisting of fruits and vegetables (not juices) has its shortcomings. Roughages, residues and other wooden elements are a burden to the digestive system. Even a healthy body with sound digestive system has the capacity of disintegrating only 35% of the ingredients from the vegetables and assimilate them. In illness, this capacity wears out. So it is possible that the body may not acquire essential substances from vegetables in sufficient quantities. That is why the use of their juices is recommended. The body is able to absorb 95% of substances contained in juices. Moreover, the healthy body and the strong teeth require a lot of time for chewing and eating fruits and vegetables which have to be consumed in large quantities to get sufficient quantity of necessary substances out of them. The result is that the body fails to acquire a necessary quantum of essential substances. To avoid all this, the use of live juices of vegetables and fruits is recommended.

Some persons complain that taking vegetable and fruit juices do not satisfy the palate and appetite. A proper combination of juices will redress this kind of complaint.

Generally if carrot-juice, apple-juice and lemon-juice each is mixed with any other juice, the result is a tasty juice. This method can be adopted when several unpalatable vegetable-juices have to be consumed.

It is not advisable to take fruit and vegetable-juices together at the same time. It is advisable to keep a gap of 3 to 4 hours between the two types of juices. Fruit juices should be taken in the first half of the day and vegetable juices should be taken in the afternoon or in the evening.

Live juices – useful to all : Vitamins, minerals and enzymes are essential for the restoration of the blood-corpuscles and the cells. They are obtained from raw vegetables, fruits and their juices. The body itself can produce certain substances, but after youth this capacity of the body wears out. So in an advanced age such food is necessary as would be digested and absorbed easily and quickly so that the process of reconstruction of the blood-corpuscles and the cells might be maintained. Fruit and vegetable juices do this important function.

These live juices are equally necessary for children and adults. Children pay attention mostly to their games and are careless about their food habits. Consequently, they do not get sufficient and proper nourishment. In these circumstances, they require nourishing food. You will hardly find a child or a youth having patience and understanding the importance of chewing food slowly while eating it. Unless fruits and vegetables are chewed profusively, the most essential elements contained in their rinds and fibres cannot be separated. This is the reason why children and adults are not benefited though they eat them in large quantities. One to one and a half kg. of vegetables and fruits might have to be taken daily in order to get the required nutrients. Who can find leisure to chew and eat such a large quantity of food? This problem has only one solution. Children and young persons should be provided with juice-diet. Juice-diet supplies all the necessary substances such as vitamins, minerals and enzymes required by the body without labour and loss of time. Thus old, adults, young and children alike require juice-diet.

Prevention of a disease is better than its cure. Children and young persons cannot get nutritious substances necessary for their body because of their improper diet and bad food habits. Owing to their undesirable habits and likings for food, the blood corpuscles and the tissue cells are destroyed instead of being reconstructed. Several vices and present unhealthy environment have worn out and weakened our children and young generation. If we want to save them from further deterioration, they should be persuaded to form the habit of taking juice-diet.

A comparison between fruit-juices and vegetable-juices : All of us would ask a question – which juices are more important in juice-diet – fruit-juices or vegetable-juices? Its answer is somewhat argumentative, because eminent dieticians have not yet come to one conclusion. The advocates of fruit-juices (Fruitarians) believe that only fruit-juices constitute an essential diet for mankind. Almost all the substances necessary for the human body can be obtained from them.

Yet, the experiments and analysis conducted so far have proved that vegetables are richer than fruits in view of their nutritious values. In a book entitled 'The Mountain Gorilla, Ecology and Behaviour' written by George B. Schaller, it is mentioned that fruits cannot supply all the elements necessary for a human body. Of course, fruits are comparatively very tasty and delicious and to extract juice from them is easy.

Only taste and flavour do not make fruits nutritious and full of all nutrients. In view of nutrients, vegetables are preferable to fruits. Considering this, a dispute over the qualities of fruits and vegetables is meaningless. We should make the balanced use of both the fruits and vegetables for health and cure of disease. Both fruits and vegetables should be considered equally beneficial to mankind. Yet it may be added that a physically fit and healthy person may rely solely on fruits but the sick, the old and children should invariably take vegetable-juices with fruit-juices.

Fruit-juices do the work of purifying blood. They cast out the toxic elements accumulated in the cells of the body. Fruits or fruit-juices increase the quantity of urine through which all toxic elements of the body are thrown out. On the other hand, raw vegetables and their juices do the work of reconstruction in the body. Vegetable-juices produce new cells in place of those that have been destroyed owing to a disease.

Those who adopt juice-diet should select varieties of fruits and vegetables. Some varieties are richer in some substances than the others. A person can get almost all the nutritious substances in proper proportion required by his body by making frequent changes in the selection of fruits and vegetables.

Fruit-juices and vegetable-juices are supplementary to each other. So those who adopt naturopathy and juice-therapy should, without any discrimination, consume juices of varied fruits and vegetables regularly.

As most of dieticians are opposed to mixing fruit-juices with vegetable-juices, it is desirable to take them separately at different times of the day. As fruit-juices are diuretic, they should not be taken in the evening or at night. The best time for taking fruit-juices is the first half of the day, but vegetable-juices can be taken at any time of the day. They can be taken in the latter half of the day also.

Juice-diet and sexual ability : A number of persons occasionally inquire whether vegetables, fruits or their juices have beneficial effects on sexual life. This question needs a detailed discussion.

2 / Juice-diet for Perfect Health

Since ancient times people have been making the use of various fruit-juices for the purpose of increasing their ability for sexual pleasure. There are references in which it is stated that the ancient Greeks used to consume cabbage-juice to increase their sexual ability. The Balkan peasants of Russia regularly drink pumpkin-juice to maintain their sexual ability till their old age. It is a common belief that there are juices of many fruits and vegetables like onion-juice, carrot-juice, etc. which contain the substances that increase sexual ability.

First of all, it is necessary to understand the scientific facts regarding sexual life. Sexual excitement depends upon two forces : (1) the mind and (2) the secretion of some glands. The prime need is the desire for sexual pleasure. When this desire arises, the brain sends a message to some endocrine glands which secrete some live chemicals (hormones) and there is sexual excitement. Thus, if there is an intense desire for sexual pleasure and, if there are a proper balance and regulation of the secretion of endocrine glands, sexual life becomes contented.

In our country, sexual life is shy and reserved and no methodical sex-education is imparted. Hence this simple, natural activity is believed to be complex.

According to the opinion of Dr. James Litham of 'Bureau of Biological Research' at Rutzers University of America, sexual ability and general health are directly related to nutrition. If food is properly planned and regulated, both sexual ability and health can be obtained and maintained easily.

Yet, many frightened people or those enticed by alluring advertisements run after medicines in order to acquire or increase sexual ability. They rely on these stimulating drugs and become mentally and financially afflicted. As a matter of fact, no medicinal herb or calx can improve sexual ability. These medicines perhaps bring a temporary sensual excitement, but in the long run they greatly damage the body. These stimulative drugs produce malefic heat in the body. The consumption of these medicines causes skin-diseases and abdominal disorders. Despite this, the manufacturers of such drugs and their dealers make a fortune out of the ignorance or anxiety of the people. Some present doctors too prescribe synthetic hormones for the treatment of sexual weakness. These doctors take the undue advantage of people's eagerness for regaining their lost sexual ability. Of course, the use of such drugs can, to certain extent, be justified only if the endocrine glands are diseased and fail to produce secretion. But in the absence of any definite cause a doctor should not prescribe such drugs even though pressed by his patient. The drugs containing synthetic hormones produce harmful side-effects.

Science now supports the belief that fruits and vegetables increase sexual ability. The Bureau of Britain has recently published a report giving information about fresh fruits and vegetables. The report supports the theory that fruit and vegetable-juices contain the elements that stimulate the desire for sensual pleasure. The report adds that in the human brain there is a part called 'limbic system' which is the source of the instincts of hunger, thirst, sex, etc. Fruit and vegetable-juices properly stimulate this 'limbic system'.

Vitamin 'A', richly contained in spinach, carrot, watermelon, mango and plums helps to transform cholesterol into active sexual hormones.

Similarly, vitamin 'B' richly contained in potatoes, banana and pumpkin plays a major role in the production of sexual hormones.

Bananas can reduce mental stress. If one is under mental stress, one's sex-hormones are adversely affected causing undesirable restriction. Bananas are rich in potassium which relieves mental stress. Consequently, there is a proper secretion of hormones.

Vitamin 'E' is also very valuable for sexual life. Vitamin 'E' in English is called 'anti-sterility' vitamin. Its deficiency causes impotence. Wheat-husk, raw vegetables, fruits, millet, sesame, etc. contain plenty of Vitamin 'E'. It is a proven fact that the intake of these substances in sufficient quantities improves sexual life.

The health of the prostate gland is important for the regulation and prolongation of sexual life. Zinc mineral is useful to keep the prostate gland active. This mineral is easily available from French beans, cucumber, onion, spinach, carrot and cabbage-juice.

As stated earlier, the addiction to tobacco, cigarettes, marijuana, liquor, etc. destroys valuable vitamins contained in the body. Fruit and vegetable-juices control this damage and help to eliminate its effects. Thus, vitamins are necessary for healthy sex-life and their best sources are fruits and vegetables.

In short, the regular consumption of fruits, vegetables and their juices produces sexual ability, improves it and also maintains it for a very long time. Moreover, these juices are free from side-effects and improve general health too.

4. HOW TO OBTAIN ALL THE NUTRIENTS FROM JUICES

Everybody desires to live a long, healthy life. His efforts are always directed towards that goal. In case he falls ill, he endeavours to get a speedy recovery from his illness. This expectation of man can be realized and his efforts can meet with success through vegetable and fruit-juices. But the important problem is how to get all the nutrients that are contained in fruit and vegetable-juices, for the recovery from disease depends on the availability of all the nutrients contained in fruit and vegetable juices.

Juices must always be fresh. Only fresh, live juices are effective for the cure of disease. Carotene (which is converted into Vitamin 'A') found in vegetables is very sensitive to oxygen in the air, e.g., if carrots are shredded and kept unused for 20 to 25 minutes, most of their vitamin 'A' is oxidized. Similarly, if lemons, oranges, mozambiques and other citrus fruits which contain vitamin 'C' are preserved for a month, about 40% of their vitamin 'C' is lost. Even a refrigerator cannot prevent this loss.

These facts emphasize that fruits and vegetables should be fresh so that all their elements can be obtained.

Another matter of importance is how to extract juice from fruits and vegetables. Fruits and vegetables should be washed, shredded or cut before extracting their juice. Then immediately they should be put into the juicer for extracting juice. In case one wants to extract juice without the help of a juicer, juice-extracting should be quick. This will save juices from being oxidized and all their nutritional elements contained in them are preserved.

Rinds and fibres of fruits and vegetables are rich sources of vitamins. So while extracting juice they should be properly crushed. However, care should be taken that juice ready for drinking does not contain fibre or rind. Juice-diet aims at getting the maximum live elements with the minimum labour by the digestive system.

To get the maximum benefits from the juices of fruits and vegetables, they must be taken fresh. Preserved juices lose their precious nutrients. It is not advisable to extract at a time the juice required for the whole day. Extract juice when required to drink.

There is a special method for drinking juice. It should not be gulped. It should be drunk slowly with a spoon or with small draughts. By this process juice gets mixed with the saliva. The digestive juices which the saliva contains help to digest sugar contained in juice. Thus, the juice which goes into the stomach is then digested within 20 to 25 minutes.

When juices are consumed for the purpose of health or cure of disease, do not add sugar, pepper or salt for taste or liking. The addition of condiments to juice is injurious to health. Furthermore, these condiments adversely affect the precious nutrients of juices. If you dislike the taste of the juice of one of the vegetables, you can add some lemon juice or any fruit-juice to it.

Canned or bottled juices are useless for those who desire to get the maximum benefits from the juice-diet because the process made on such juices and their preservation destroy almost all their live nutrients. Furthermore, certain harmful preservatives and chemicals are added to them. Canned or bottled juices are referred to as 'fresh'. But it signifies that the juices have been extracted from fresh fruits. Thus, juices, even if extracted from fresh fruits, lose their live nutrients when they are preserved. Hence we should not mistake such juices for fresh.

Most of the canned or bottled juices are mixed with chemicals such as sugar, salt and others. Consequently, their original colour, taste, flavour, etc. are retained and spoilage is prevented. The most commonly used preservatives for canned or bottled juices are benzoic acid, sulphuric acid or sorbic acid. All these chemicals are injurious to health. Heating is one of the principal processes made on fruit-juices for the purposes of preservation. Heating destroys most of the nutrients contained in fruit-juices.

From the point of view of vitamin content fresh and tinned juices are miles apart. That can be seen from two examples. The vitamin 'C' content in fresh carrot-juice is 8 mg, while that in canned juice is only 2 mg. Similarly, the vitamin 'C' content in fresh spinach-juice is 51 mg, while that in canned juice is only 14 mg.

By consuming canned or bottled juices, chemicals contained in them would perhaps cause ulcer, kidney-diseases, dental carries, cancer, etc. So, if freshly extracted juices of seasonal fruits and vegetables are consumed, they will be beneficial to health and cure of disease.

Method to extract juice : First of all fresh fruits and vegetables should be purchased. They should be of good quality. It should be remembered that preserved or stocked fruits and vegetables have already lost several of their essential vitamins. Fruits should always be ripe but not overripe. Fruits ripened artificially with the help of chemicals should never be selected. Fruits and vegetables grown with the help of natural compost manure are superior in quality to those grown with the help of chemical fertilizers. Normally, it is better to have vegetables grown in one's own farm or close to one's own house.

Electric juicer is the best instrument for extracting juice from fresh fruits and vegetables, because it also crushes the fibres and rinds of vegetables and fruits and pour out their rich elements into the juice. From this point of view there is no alternative to electric juicer. A good quality-juicer costs about a thousand rupees. In its absence, one can manually extract juice from fruits and vegetables by crushing and mashing them.

Before extracting juice from fruits or vegetables, they should be washed out and cut into small pieces. If their rind is not very hard and is edible, it should not be peeled off because some of the rich elements are contained in it. Immediately put the shredded pieces into juicer and extract juice. If necessary, pour some water Filter the juice to avoid fibres. Juices of fruits and vegetables should be used immediately after they have been extracted. Preserved or stocked juices come into contact with oxygen in the air. This oxidation of juices destroys most of their precious vitamins. According to expert dieticians, one should 'eat' juice instead of drinking it. Juice should not be swallowed hastily but taken slowly draught by draught.

After extracting juice, the juicer should be thoroughly washed and cleaned with warm water otherwise bacteria are produced in the juicer and they mix with juice when extracted next time.

It is true that a middle class family cannot afford to have a juicer which costs about a thousand rupees but ultimately it proves economical. Many persons spend money after medicines instead of taking juice for the cure of disease. But money invested in a juicer is more economical and proper than money spent on medicines.

Quantity of juice to be taken daily : Almost all dieticians say, "The more juice you drink, the quicker will be the results and benefits." Some experts inform us that there is no harm involved and only benefit to be derived from taking large quantities of fresh juice. The consumption of fruit-juices in large quantities has no ill-effects. Dr. Henry Sherman, an eminent scientist and dietician, is of the opinion that the more you drink the juices of various fruits and vegetables regularly with planning, the quicker will be the relief from diseases.

When a person goes on a raw vegetable or fruit-juice diet, it is usually because he has abused his body for 50 to 60 or even more years. To undo the harm of wrong eating and wrong living for all those years, large quantities of juices are required. Those with wide experience and who have conquered diseases including terminal malignancies, state that five litres of juice per day and even more is not too much. But this quantity is for those who desire to live solely on a juice-diet for longer time. In general, a partaker of juice-diet should drink minimum two to three litres of juice per day for improving and maintaining his health.

Half or three quarters of litre of juice should be taken five to six times a day, with an interval of two to two and a half hours. One who has a good health and has adopted juice-diet to maintain it should also take at least a litre of juice of various fruits and vegetables per day. A partaker of raw food and dried fruits need not take large quantities of juices.

The juices of ginger, onions and green turmeric being highly concentrated and strong are restricted to not more than 20-25 ml per day.

A table spoonful of garlic juice is sufficient for a day. Similarly, the consumption of coriander and basil juices should not exceed 20-25 ml per day. Water is required to be added while extracting certain juices.

A person who decides to live solely on only juice-diet in order to get rid of certain chronic and dangerous diseases should take daily 5 to 6 litres of juices of various fruits and vegetables. Juice-diet then prevents physical energy from being consumed in digestion. Later, after the health is improved, he can start taking raw food, dried fruits, etc. with a gradual decrease in the quantity of juices. The daily maintenance quantum of juices is one to one and a half litres.

The time-limit of juice-diet : A partaker of juice-diet would naturally ask a question : 'How long should juice-diet be continued?' There is another question also : 'Can anyone live on juice-diet for a long time?' Expert dieticians with wide experience agree that a person can live his entire life on juice-diet and wheat grass juice and yet maintain health and energy.

Then, how can we obtain carbohydrates, fats, protein, sugar and other various constituents of food necessary for the body? Proteins and sugar may be obtained from juices, but it is not feasible to get fats from a juice-diet. Vitamins, minerals and enzymes are available from juices.

According to one expert opinion, juice-diet cannot satisfy protein requirement of the body throughout the life. Juice-diet is also costly. In our country, fruits and vegetables are not easily and cheaply available. Furthermore, it is a characteristic of human nature that man wants varieties. He will be tired of living on only juice-diet, leaving off tasty and delicious meals.

Considering all the reasons and conditions mentioned above, the time-limit of and discretion in the use of juice-diet can be determined as follows :

1. Prolonged juice-diet is necessary for relief from chronic and dangerous diseases.
2. After the cure of disease, there should be a gradual decrease in the quantity of juice-diet and raw food should be included in the diet.
3. Cooked food can be taken once or twice a week, especially for satisfying the palate.
4. If one wants to give rest to the digestive system and save the physical energy, one can take juice-diet according to one's need.
5. If you want to keep the body and the mind ever healthy and active, a combination of juice-diet with raw or cooked food is desirable because it serves two purposes– health and satisfaction of the palate.
6. Juice-diet taken for a week or a fortnight once or twice a year cleanses the body and cures minor diseases.

7. Juice-diet should be combined with raw food, sprouted pulses, grains, dried fruits, etc. for the maintenance of good health.

'Juice-fasting' means to live purely on juices. One cannot live the whole life only on juice-diet or juice-fasting. It is true that, if you take fruit and vegetable-juices throughout life, you can live. But permanent juice-fasting excessively weakens the digestive system, the teeth, the muscles and other organs. Therefore, one should not resolve to live on juice-diet alone for the whole life.

Nethertheless, it should be remembered that, if juice-diet is adopted for the cure of disease, it should be continued in a limited quantity even after the disease has been cured. After the relief from disease, one should not be careless to the body, for carelessness to the body is injurious to health. Juice-diet is a rejuvenator of the body and bestower of health and vitality. If one continues taking it regularly in a fixed quantity, one's life will be happy, peaceful, efficient and healthy.

---

5. JUICE-FASTING

Those who have accepted and adopted juices and raw food as their diet may naturally ask how long the diet should be continued after the body has become healthy and the disease is cured. The question is important and needs a detailed discussion.

To observe fast for religious purposes is our age-old tradition and belief. The purpose of observing fast is scientific. Fasting aims at giving rest to the digestive system. During the period of fasting, no food is taken. Sometimes, a fruit-diet is allowed. But today, the definition of fruit-diet is perverted. Instead of fruits, many other items are taken. This cannot really be called fasting and this type of 'fasting' gives no benefit to the body.

Juice-fasting is an effective and scientific method for giving real benefits to the body and the health. In this kind of fasting, nothing except fruit and vegetable-juices is taken. Many expert dieticians give great importance to this kind of fasting.

The obvious purpose of juice-fasting is to regain health by giving rest to the digestive system. Juice-diet eliminates the toxic and inorganic substances and bacteria from the body. As juice without roughage and fibres is easily digestible, the body has not to work hard for its absorption and assimilation. Juice begins to get absorbed in the body within 20-25 minutes after it is taken. Consequently, the body begins to acquire immediately the vitamins which increase the resistance power of the body against diseases. Besides, the mineral salts contained in juice neutralize acidic elements in the blood. Then why should we not take the benefit of juices which supply the body without labour the elements necessary for the cure of disease?

During juice-fasting, toxic substances in the body begin

44

to burn and this burning supplies heat to the body. Though the body has an accumulation of fats and carbohydrates, the body has a nature to burn first toxic substances. The reason for this process is that though the juices contain vitamins, minerals and enzymes in abundance, the heat-giving substances are in meagre proportion. During fasting, the combustion of accumulated stock of toxic substances automatically supplies the required heat to the body.

The excretory process of the body is stimulated during juice-fasting. Undesirable elements in the body are eliminated through the kidneys, the skin and the lungs. During the preliminary stages of juice-fasting, there is foul-breathing, urine is dark; and the body perspires profusely. But soon a stage is reached when the body becomes purified. Thereafter, breathing, urine, perspiration attain their original condition.

According to researches made by 'The Caleolinska Institute of Stockholm', the world-famous medical research institute, juice-fasting is completely safe and it should be widely publicized.

Before juice-fasting is commenced, a two-or three-day 'water-fast' is beneficial. An expert's guidance is necessary for the selection of fruits and vegetables for the cure of a particular disease. (See part 3 of this book for further information.). Begin fasting with a small quantity of juices. Gradually, increase the quantity. On the first day, take 250 ml of juices five times at the interval of three hours. Thus the total quantity of juices to be taken on the first day will be 1250 ml. On the second day take 300 ml of juice each time. Begin taking juice at seven in the morning. The last intake should be at seven in the evening. Gradually increase the quantity every day. After eight days a person having good digestion will be able to take more than 600 ml of juice each time. Thus the quantity of juices which he will take during the whole day will be 5 to 10 litres. If one feels heaviness in the stomach, it means that the quantity of juices taken is more than required. In such cases, the quantity should be decreased.

Those who want to consume more juice should reduce the interval between the two intakes and take juice seven to eight times a day.

One can continue juice-fasting for one and a half to two months. But during that time, it is possible that some symptoms like foul-breathing, headache, stomachache, insomnia, fever, bodyache, swelling of gums, etc. may arise. These symptoms, in fact, are the processes for eliminating toxic substances inhabited in the body. It is not a matter of worry. One is likely to lose some weight but one should not worry about the lost pounds. These symptoms will disappear gradually and the body will be completely cleansed.

One should strictly observe the following instructions during juice-fasting :
1. Take complete rest except, if desired, walking for a short distance in the morning.
2. One can walk for a short distance in the evening also.
3. Avoid the work which involves physical exertion.
4. Leave off anxiety and hurry. Live delightfully.
5. Have full faith in juice-fasting and be an optimist in your experiment for the improvement of health.
6. Abandon smoking and taking tea, coffee, cold drinks, alcohol, etc.

The way in which juice-fasting is terminated is also very important. The success or failure of juice-fasting depends on the post-fasting follow-up. The purpose of juice-fasting will not be served if its termination is improper. On the day of breaking the fast, juice should be taken only three times a day i.e., in the morning, at noon and in the evening. Ripe fruits without roughage and fibres should be taken in between intervals. On the second day, fruits and boiled vegetables without spices should be taken. On the third day, some milk and nuts should be taken in addition to fruits and vegetables. Begin taking sprouted pulses and food-grains on the fourth day. Then gradually start taking the usual diet. Juices in certain quantities should be continued to maintain health gained during juice-fasting.

In short, at the time of breaking juice-fasting, the following instructions should be observed :

1. Stay peacefully and delightfully.
2. Do not start eating excessive food after juice-fasting.
3. After juice-fasting is completed let a few days pass before taking the usual diet.
4. There should be a gradual increase in the quantity of food.
5. Chew properly the food you take.
6. Even after the termination of juice-fasting, some quantity of juice should be taken regularly.

Protein on a juice-diet : We have formed a firm belief that the human body and cells are constructed out of proteins and so we must invariably have proteins in our diet. Then a perennial question is : 'Will there be a protein-deficiency in the body if only juice-diet is adopted?'

It is true that protein is very essential to the body. It plays a very important role in the growth and development of the body. But the conviction that the body cannot do without protein even for some time is erroneous. One who lives on a total raw juice diet worries about protein-deficiency; but that worry can be allayed by the following expert opinions :

1. Dr. L. H. Newber of the University of Michigan in America has made experiments to observe the effects of protein-deficiency in food on the body. He observes that protein as an energy and fuel-giving element is not a satisfactory constituent of food. The excess of protein would perhaps damage the kidneys.

2. According to the distinguished physiological chemist, Dr. Russell Chittenden of Yale University, the daily amount of protein should be as low as 50 grams. This amount is sufficient for maintaining health, endurance and working power of the individual. Even a meatless diet can be a balanced and complete diet.

3. Dr. H. E. Kirschner of America gave only carrot-juice to a very weak woman suffering from neurasthenia, jaundice and kidney-stone. The woman gained 70 pounds. Thus Dr. Kirschner proved that the health of the individual and his working power can be maintained without even milk, ghee, butter, meat, etc. which contain protein.

4. After having done research for many years, Dr. N. W. Petty of England has proved that the Chlorophyll in green vegetables contains protein of a high quality. Those who consume green vegetables in sufficient amount need not worry about protein.

5. According to Dr. William C. Ritz of Northwestern University, a daily intake of 20–35 grams of protein is sufficient.

6. During the famous 'Fast March' organized in Sweden, it was observed that the persons who had not taken protein at all had maintained a usual and steady protein contents in their blood.

We should not give undue importance to protein required for the body. It is true that protein is indispensable to the body; but protein can be procured from even a small quantity of sprouted food-grains. Even fruit and vegetable juices do contain some amount of proteins.

Following is the chart showing protein contents of different fruits and vegetables :

Fruits/Vegetables	Amount of Protein Contents
Cherry	0.4 gm/100 gm
Apple	0.2 gm/100 gm
Beet	1.6 gm/100 gm
Garlic	6.2 gm/100 gm
Peas	3.4 gm/100 gm
Spinach	3.2 gm/100 gm
Carrot	1.1 gm/100 gm
French beans	1.9 gm/100 gm
Cabbage	1.3 gm/100 gm
Cauliflower	2.7 gm/100 gm
Onion	1.5 gm/100 gm
Tomato	1.1 gm/100 gm

The above list shows that one can find substantial quantities of protein in fruit and vegetable juices provided the amount of juices is substantial. One who takes raw food in addition to juice-diet gets sufficient proteins from sprouted pulses.

The protein in live fresh juices contains its full allotment of different types of enzymes and, thus, is completely assimilable, whereas the protein in cooked food, meat or milk is impaired and its assimilability is doubtful.

Thus, one should rest assured that living on only a juice-diet causes no protein deficiency.

———————

3 / Juice-diet for Perfect Health

6. TEN IMPORTANT COMMANDMENTS FOR JUICE-DIET

'Diet is health, diet is medicine,' so said Socrates several hundred years back.

Those who take to juice-diet should follow the invaluable instructions given below :

1. The purpose of juice-diet should be distinctly determined. Whether juice-diet is adopted for the purpose of maintaining health or getting relief from disease should be very clear.

2. The intake of juice-diet should be regular. If the purpose of taking juice-diet is to get rid of virulent and chronic diseases, juice-diet should be followed systematically and with all earnestness.

3. A fixed quantity of juice should be taken at predetermined fixed hours regularly every day.

4. A variety in fruits and vegetables is desirable. If the partaker of juice-diet intends to get relief from specific diseases, the selection of fruits and vegetables should be strictly under the guidance of an expert dietician.

5. In order to preserve its useful and live elements, juice should be taken fresh immediately after it has been extracted. It should be sipped by draughts. A quick swallowing of juice does not give expected results.

6. If raw food, salad or nuts are taken with the juice-diet, juice should be taken some time before the taking of these substances so that the enzymes contained in juice may help digestion.

7. A partaker of juice-diet should always drink juice with a delightful mind. Juice taken with full faith and hope is more beneficial.

50

8. During the period of juice-diet, sometimes the toxic elements concealed in the body try to find their way out through different processes of elimination like vomitting, headache, fever, etc. These symptoms are not much to be worried about. The patient should continue juice-diet without any apprehension, because these symptoms are short-lived and disappear of their own.

9. There are several other experiments which help the process of elimination of toxic elements from the body. In costive conditions enemas can be taken for eradication of accumulated stools in the intestine. Hot-water bath or vapour-bath would hasten the process of elimination of toxic elements.

10. A complete rest is recommended during the period of juice-diet. Though hard work and exercises are contraindicated during juice-fasting, light yogasanas and a short-distance walk are permissible.

The latest Juice-diet researches : The preventive and curative value of raw food has excited the scientists all over the world so much that a number of centres and hospitals are now conducting experiments on this subject. Here are a few examples of some of the latest researches.

Dr. D. C. Hare of the Royal Free Hospital in England put a group of arthritic patients on a diet consisting purely of raw food and juices for two weeks and then a predominantly raw food diet for several more weeks. Practically all of the patients began to feel better within one to four weeks, with marked improvement continuing thereafter.

J. F. Kinderheilk, a research scholar, states that the raw food diet is of immense value in avitaminosis, nephritis, diabetes and chronic constipation.

Dr. W. Heupe of the University Medical Polyclinic in Frankfurt reports that a raw food diet aids in the treatment of diarrhoea of children, in heart and kidney diseases, and in obesity and diabetes.

I. Kanai, a researcher from the University of Berlin, carefully studied and examined the effect of raw and cooked vegetarian diets on the process of oxidation taking place in the body. His experiments clearly showed that oxidation was impaired by cooked vegetarian foods. On a raw food diet the urinary output of nitrogen was greater, indicating better absorption of food-elements in the blood.

Dr. M. Kuratsune of Kyushu University in Japan also tested the effects of raw and cooked vegetarian diets on the body. It was discovered that exclusive cooked food tended to create anemia, which cleared up when some of the cooked food was replaced by raw food. Many other disorders, which had failed to respond to the conventional medical care, improved considerably on the raw diet.

Dr. Joseph Evers of Germany has treated nearly 1,000 cases of **Multiple Sclerosis** with diets which included only raw food. The success enjoyed by Dr. Evers in the treatment of Multiple Sclerosis is in itself the greatest documentation in the world for the value of the raw food diet. No other doctor anywhere in the world claims beneficial treatment for Multiple Sclerosis. For over 10 years people from every part of the world have been going to Dr. Evers for the treatment of this disease.

In the present time, the work of Dr. Kristine Nolfi of Denmark regarding raw food is unique. She recovered from cancer after treating herself with an exclusive raw food diet. After that, she opened an institution called 'Humlegaarden' which gave such type of treatment. This system of healing and treatment gave her unexpected success and credit. Inspired by this, Dr. Nolfi has written a book on raw food, which is worth reading and meditating upon.

Dr. Nolfi's own life-story is also very interesting. In 1940–41, Dr. Nolfi was diagnosed as having cancer but she refused treatment by X-ray, radium or surgery. Because of her refusal to accept established, approved medical treatment she was thwarted and persecuted until she discontinued her medical practice. She shifted to Humlegaarden where she successfully treated herself with an exclusive raw food. She recovered from cancer. Then she opened an establishment at Humlegaarden and treated many cancer and other patients with raw food. About 1,000 patients visit the sanatorium annually. Not only patients but all the members of the hospital staff also live purely on raw food and enjoy good health. Dr. Nolfi gives a great deal of credit to raw garlic and raw potatoes which, she claims, are key vegetables in the success of raw food diet.

If raw food can bestow such unimaginable benefits, why should people unnecessarily suffer from ailments and rot in diseases? There is no doubt that 'raw food and juices' is the shortest and simplest way to perfect health.

PART 2

CONTENTS AND QUALITIES OF FRUITS AND VEGETABLES

1. APPLE

'An apple a day keeps the doctor away.'

— The old proverb

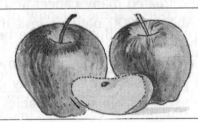

Introduction : The early home of the apples is believed to be the Caucasus Mountains. It is now grown in all the parts of the world. It has been known to India for over many centuries. Apples are available in abundance in the months of August and September, although now they are grown all the year round. The apple is considered as one of the best fruits.

Qualities : The apple has a sweet-sour taste. It is constipating, nourishing and easily digestible. It helps to quench thirst. It appeases bile and windiness, cures dysentery and strengthens intestines. Its pectin content relieves cough and helps in eliminating toxic elements from the body. It is very useful in decreasing the acidity in the stomach. It vitalizes the heart, the brain, the liver and the stomach. It works as an appetizer and improves the quality of blood.

Analysis of Contents

Water	85.9%
Protein	0.3%
Fat	0.1%
Carbohydrates	9.5%

Minerals	0.4%
Calcium	0.01%
Phosphorus	0.02%
Iron	1.7 mg/100 grams
Vitamin 'B'	40 I. U/100 grams
Vitamin 'C'	Trace

It also contains a small amount of copper.

Use : Fresh apple juice is very convenient for the consumption. Of course, some quantity of apples can be masticated and eaten raw. But to get the benefits of more nutrients fresh apple juice recommended.

Benefits : Supporting the medicinal qualities of the apple, the American Medical Association has stated that the apple is very useful in the cases of children's diarrhoea. Though the apple has laxative qualities, the pectin in it checks diarrhoea.

Dr. J. H. Kellogg, the celebrated dietarian of Battle Creek, U.S.A. is of the opinion that the apple is an excellent disinfectant for the stomach and intestines. He further states that it is a valuable remedy in jaundice and in cases in which the kidneys and the liver are diseased.

It is also recommended as a good remedy for gout and arthritis.

Fresh apple-juice is most wholesome when taken with honey.

Apple-juice gives relief in the weakness of the nervous system, kidney-stone, acidity, indigestion, headache, biliousness, asthma and dysentery.[1]

The slight acid content of the apple also exerts an antiseptic influence upon the germs present in the mouth and teeth, when it is taken by chewing sufficiently. It may therefore be looked upon as a natural protector of the teeth and hence should be taken in all tooth troubles.

***

---

1. Jadu Nath Ganguli, M. B – Dyspepsia, p. 24, Banaras

2. BEETROOT

"Beet juice can cure cancer."

— *Dr. Firenczi, Hungary :*

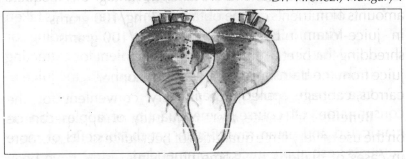

Introduction : The native home of the beet is the Mediterranean area and the South-Western Asia. The beetroot has been used as food for the last 2,000 years. The early Romans and the Greeks used to consume it profusely. The old Greeks looked upon the beet as being good for cooling the blood. The beet is a bulbous root. It resembles a top. It is of two colours–red-violet and white.

Qualities : The beetroot is somewhat hard to digest. It is oily, cool, nutritious and a bile-controller. It improves the quality of the blood. It reddens and vitalizes the body. The betaine content of the beet helps in cleansing the stomach and the intestine.

Analysis of Contents

Water	83.8%
Protein	1.7%
Fat	0.1%
Carbohydrates	13.6%
Calcium	0.20%
Phosphorus	0.06%
Vitamin 'B$_1$'	210 microgrammes/100 gm
Vitamin 'B$_2$'	90 microgrammes/100 gm
Nicotinic acid	0.4 mg.
Vitamin 'C'	8.8 mg/100 gm

Use : The beetroot is used as a salad. We in India rarely use the beet, but in foreign countries the beet-juice is widely used and its unique benefits are taken advantage of. Adequate amounts of nutrients can be obtained only when beet is taken in juice-form. Juice can be extracted by pounding or shredding the beet. A juicer is very convenient for extracting juice from the beet. Beet-juice can be mixed with the juice of carrots, cabbage, mango or papaya.

Benefits : In France, there have been many experiments on the use of very large quantities of beet-juice to aid recovery in cases of malignancy. Some promising results have been reported. In Germany, beet-juice is available in bottles. It is widely used as a powerful restorative during convalescence.

In 1946, a German naturopath Kunstmann was successful in curing a number of cancer-patients with beet-juice. Thereafter, in 1950, Dr. Firenczi from Hungary successfully treated a patient of malignant tumour with beet-juice. It was noted that beet-juice had a beneficial effect on other ailments also. Many patients gained weight by consuming beet-juice. At Sorna´in Hungary the experiments on this beet-therapy are still in progress. In this therapy, the patient is supported on water fast for first two days. Then for a few days the patient is given fruit-juices. In the third stage, he is given a mixture of 250 grams of beet-juice and 250 grams of carrot-juice. This regimen is then continued throughout the treatment period.

Beet-juice is harmless and beneficial. As it is rejuvenating, it is effective in every type of weakness. It also purifies the blood and brings redness to the body.

***

3. BEL *(Bilifal)*

"As a remedy for bowel complaints, diarrhoea and chronic dysentery, the juice of bel fruit has no equal."

— *Dr. Devaprosad Sanyal, Calcutta*

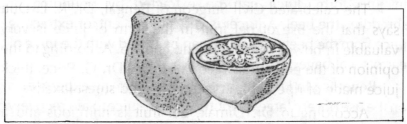

Introduction : 'Bel' is a native of India. From time immemorial it has been regarded as a medicinal herb. It is round in shape and resembles a wood-apple. It is of the normal ball-size. It is sweet in taste. It contains a lot of seeds.

Qualities : Bel is sweet, light, digestive, a kindler of gastric fire and slightly constipating. It destroys intestinal worms, stops nausea, vomitting and relieves cramps of stomach-muscles. In fact, the Ayurveda considers it 'Tridosh-har' i.e. a remedy for the three systemic disturbances viz. cough, wind and bile.

Analysis of Contents

Water	84.00%
Protein	0.7%
Fat	0.7%
Carbohydrate	16.2%
Tannin	9.00 to 20.00%[1]
Vitamin 'C'	7.6 mg./100 gm.

Besides these, it also contains small amount of vitamin 'B_1', vitamin 'B_2' niacin, calcium, phosphorus and iron.

Use : The pulp of the ripe bel may be taken directly or it may be taken in its juice-form.

1. I.H.Burkill, F.L.S.–A Dictionary of the Economic Products of the Malay Peninsula, p. 37.

Benefits : The medicinal value of bel is principally dependent upon the tannin it contains. In digestive disorders and chronic dysentery, bel is regarded as an invaluable remedy.[1]

The celebrated Civil Surgeon of Bengal, Dr. R. L. Dutt says that the use of bel fruit in the form of juice is very valuable in bowel complaints and cholera. According to the opinion of the eminent surgeon of Bihar, Dr. G. Price, thick juice made of ripe bel fruit is the best and surest laxative.

According to Dr. Dimak, bel fruit is nutritious and a blood-purifier. 50 mg. of the juice of bel fruit mixed with warm water and sugar, two-three times a day helps to eradicate blood-impurities.

***

4. BITTER GOURD *(Karela)*

"A glass of bitter gourd juice taken on an empty stomach is a sure beneficial remedy for jaundice."

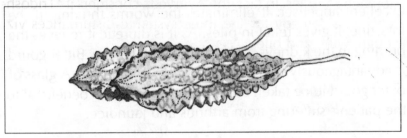

Introduction : Bitter gourds are one · of the Indians' favourite vegetables. Those who cherish bitter gourds buy them at any price when there is the season of bitter gourds. The bitter gourd is usually five to six inches long.

Qualities : Bitter gourds are bitter in taste, stimulant of gastric fire, light for digestion, warm, purgative, soothing and conducive to digestion. They are excellent appetiser and cure

1. Devaprosad Sanyal – Vegetable Drugs of India, p. 116, Calcutta

cough, windiness, blood impurities, fever, worms, bile, anaemia and leucoderma.

Analysis of Contents

Water	92.4%
Protein	11.6%
Fat	0.2%
Carbohydrates	4.2%
Minerals	0.8%
Calcium	0.02%
Phosphorus	0.07%
Iron	2.2 mg/100 gm
Vitamin 'A'	210 I. U./100 gm
Vitamin 'B'	24 I. U/100 gm
Vitamin 'C'	88 mg/100 gm

Use : A glass of bitter gourd juice taken on an empty stomach is immediately beneficial to health

Benefits : Bitter gourd juice purifies blood. It is an excellent appetiser. It eliminates the worms thriving in the intestine. It gives relief in piles. As it is diuretic it relieves the burning in the kidneys. It dissolves kidney-stone. Bitter gourd is advantageously effective in the cases of diabetes. A glass of bitter gourd juice taken on an empty stomach is beneficial to the patients suffering from arthritis and jaundice.

* * *

5. CABBAGE

"The vitamin 'U' contained in cabbage is a sure remedy for duodenal and gastric ulcers."

— *Dr. Garneth Cheney, California*

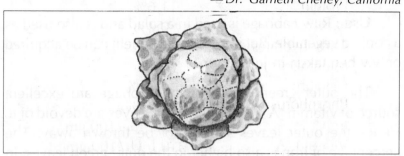

Introduction : Cabbage is considered as a leafy vegetable. It was brought to India from Europe and has become very popular. It grows in abundance in winter.

Qualities : Cabbage is delicious, vitalizing, pungent, bitter, cool, digestive and light. It kindles gastric fire and is good for the heart. To some extent it produces windiness. It is useful in cough, bile, leucoderma, coughing and impurities of the blood.

Analysis of Contents

Water	90.2%
Protein	1.8%
Fat	0.1%
Carbohydrates	6.3%
Minerals	0.6%
Calcium	0.03%
Phosphorus	0.05%
Iron	0.8 mg/100 gm
Vitamin 'A'	2000 I. U./100 gm
Vitamin 'B$_1$'	60 microgram/100 gm
Vitamin 'B$_2$'	30 microgram/100 gm
Niacin	0.4 mg/100 gm
Vitamin 'C'	124 mg/100 gm

One of the reasons for which cabbage is esteemed is its ascorbic acid (vitamin 'C') content. Nearly one-third of the day's allowance of vitamin 'C' may be secured from only one cup of raw chopped cabbage.

Use : Raw cabbage is used in a salad and is also used as a cooked vegetable. But its medicinal benefit can be acquired only when taken in juice-form.

The outer green leaves of the cabbage are excellent source of vitamin 'A'. The inner white leaves are devoid of it. Hence the outer leaves should not be thrown away. The percentage of iron is also higher in the outer green leaves. In cooking cabbage, every attempt should be made to keep the cooking time at a minimum. Excessive heat treatment of cabbage is destructive to its vitamin 'B' and vitamin 'C' contents.[2] Under no circumstances should the water, in which the cabbage is boiled, be thrown away. It contains many nutrients such as vitamin 'C', calcium, iron, phosphorus and magnesium.[3]

Benefits : According to the opinion of Dr. Garneth Cheney, M. D. of Stanford University School of Medicine, California, the cabbage contains a new vitamin which cures gastric and duodenal ulcers. This factor in food is called vitamin 'U'. Dr. Garneth Cheney has successfully applied cabbage in the treatment of 65 patients who were suffering from these ulcers. This anti-peptic ulcer factor is destroyed when cabbage is boiled.[4] As cabbage furnishes sufficient assimilable iron, it is also very useful in the treatment of anaemia.

---

1. Michael G. Wohl, M. D. Dietotherapy, p. 947, Saunders Co., Philadelphia
2. Alida Francis Patter–Practical Dietetics, p. 652, New York
3. Dr. James S. Melester, M. D.–Guide to Health, p. 114.
4. Oliver E. Byed, M. D.–Health Instruction Handbook-1951, p. 33-34, Stanford Uni. Press, California

Dr. O'Dell and his co-workers submitted a paper at the fifth International Congress of Nutrition in Washington. The paper reported that the addition of cabbage to a completely balanced feed for female guinea pigs produced an appreciable effect on their growth and a much improved resistance to infection from the virulent mouse-typhus. Dr. Rudat also found the claim to be substantial.

Some unknown dietary factors in cabbage are yet not identified but their presence in cabbage is certain. Dr. Cheney had treated ulcer patients with 450 ml of cabbage juice each at the intervals of a few hours every day. Their pain subsided only in five days and healing occurred by the fourteenth day. One cannot expect gratifying results even within seven weeks with medical treatment in vogue.

Dr. Hannon wrote to the American Medical Association Journal with examples of the good results obtained in patients with digestive conditions of long-standing, that had proved resistant to normal treatment, by giving raw cabbage juice. It should be noted that initially Dr. Hannon had his own doubts about the efficacy of the cabbage treatment. He had used cabbage as the last resort for experimental purposes.

Cabbage is found very effective in conditions such as arthritis, neurasthenia, pyorrhoea, indigestion, anaemia, defective vision and obesity. Looking to the above qualities and effectiveness of cabbage, eminent Indian physicians have named it 'Dalamalini'.

* * *

6. CARROT

"Carrot-juice contains carotene (pro-vitamin 'A') which is very beneficial to the eyes."

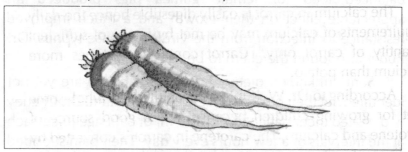

Introduction : It is said that the early home of the carrot was Kashmir, the western Himalayas, Europe, Northern Asia, Abyssinia and Northern Africa. Now it has spread all over the world. The carrot is an edible bulbous root. It varies in size from four-five inches to ten-twelve inches and it is orange-red in colour. The variety known as Delhi carrot is good and delicious.

Qualities : The carrot is sweet, warm, pleasant, stimulant of gastric fire, dry, appetiser, diuretic, constipating and to some extent bitter. It gives relief in fistula, worms and dysentery. It eradicates windiness and cough. If taken in excess, it increases bile.

Analysis of Contents

Water	86.00%
Protein	0.9%
Fat	0.2%
Carbohydrates	10.7%
Calcium	0.08%
Phosphorus	0.53%
Iron	1.5 mg/100 gm
Carotene (Vitamin 'A')	2000 to 4300 I. U./100 gm
Vitamin 'B'	60 I. U./100 gm

Besides all these, it contains vitamin 'C' and vitamin 'D', niacin. Pyrodoxine, folic acid, biotin, pantothenic acid in minute quantities, and the minerals potassium, sodium, magnesium, copper, etc. in small amounts.

The calcium in carrot is easily digestible hence the daily requirements of calcium may be met by intake of sufficient quantity of carrot only.[1] Carrot contains six times more calcium than potato.

According to Dr. W. Kubler, carrot juice is a wholesome diet for growing children because it is a good source of carotene and calcium. The carotene in carrot is converted by the liver into vitamin A and is also stored therein.

Use : Carrot-juice is easily extracted with the help of a juicer. Juice can also be extracted by shredding it minutely and pounding it. The middle yellow part of carrot (root) should be discarded. Carrot can be eaten also by chewing it well.

Benefits : Carrots eaten by chewing cleanse and strengthen the teeth. Grated carrots mixed with a small amount of salt have beneficial effects on eczema. Carrots are an excellent food for maintaining health of the eyes. Carrots contain a hormone known as tocokinin. This is an insulin-like compound which has been proved useful in diabetes.[2]

A well-known American magazine 'Saturday Evening Post' quotes the following experiment in its isssue of May 1982. The American National Cancer Institute and the National Heart Lung and Blood Institute jointly are conducting experiment on 22,000 American citizens. These people are being given raw carrots and vegetables. Four crore rupees have been sanctioned for this experiment tentatively. One can get easily convinced about the importance of carrot and juice-diet by the huge amount being spent by the

1. J. H. Kellogg, M. D. – The New Dietetics, p. 304, Modern Publishing Co., Washington
2. Houser and Berg – The Dictionary of Food

scientists on the experiments concerned. These experiments will be conducted for four years and after that results will be known.

Dr. Metchnikoff of Russia has proved by experiments that carrot has insecticidal properties. It destroys harmful bacteria thriving in the intestine.[1] One gets relief from enteritis with the help of carrot-juice. It also heals intestinal ulcers.[2]

The carrot is diuretic in action. It may therefore be used in nephritis as a food medicine. It is also very helpful in scanty urination.

Carrot-juice eliminates unwanted uric acid from the blood and is, therefore, very helpful for gout-patients. It is regarded as a remedy for gallstone troubles, liver diseases, tuberculosis and scanty menstruation.

Experiments have proved that carrot has an ample amount of vitamin 'E'. Eminent dietarians have regarded this vitamin as very useful for the body. Vitamin 'E' is believed to contain an antisterility factor.

Experiments made on animals show that vitamin 'E' increases their procreative capacity. Cancer cells cannot thrive in the blood because of vitamin 'E'. Animals fed on the diet containing sufficient vitamin 'E' develop resistance to cancer. Experiments regarding this have been made on man and a good deal of success has been accomplished. It has been established that carrot juice has a property that checks cancer. It is natural that the juice that can treat a dreadful disease like cancer successfully can cure other disease as well.

---

1. Council of Scientific and Industrial Research–The Wealth of India, Vol. III, p. 21, New Delhi
2. An Indian Dietarian –Food and Nutrition in India, p. 182, Calcutta

THE MIRACLES OF CARROT-JUICE

(1)

Here is a case which shows the miracle of carrot-juice. It has happened in Cansass, U. S. A. In this case carrot-juice had saved a child from dying and given him new life. The child's mother herself narrates the exciting experience.

"At the time of his birth my son was very healthy. His progress continued without any hurdle. When he was about fourteen months old, he fell ill. He suffered from hysterical attacks (fits). He remained unconscious for about eight hours. Following our doctor's advice we shifted him to the hospital. Immediately a medicine was injected in his thigh. Thereafter he did not suffer hysterical attacks, but remained unconscious for three days.

"After a week, the hospital doctors informed that my son was free from disease and that we could return home. They advised me to give my son nutritious food. We followed their advice with care and perseverance. Despite this, my son kept falling ill at the intervals of a few days. Occasionally he suffered from hysterical fits.

"He was mentally broken. He was subsequently examined by more than twelve doctors. Each of them diagnosed differently. In spite of being given the best nutritious food, he was losing weight.

"When my son was two years old, it seemed to me that his health had started improving. But that outward appearance turned out to be deceptive. After having examined him, the doctor stated that he was suffering from enteritis. We were shocked. My son cried continuously. He was unable to eat anything. His body had become allergic to animal foods including milk. Whatever he ate was not digested. There was no usual evacuation of his bowels. The presence of mucous and blood in his faeces worried us.

"When he was two and half years old, his physical condition had worsened so much that he was unable even to change side by himself. He appeared like a skeleton of bones and skin. His weight was now only 16 pounds. The hope that he would survive had dwindled. Most of the doctors came to the conclusion that the boy had been suffering from intestinal tuberculosis and there was no hope for his recovery. They opined that even if the boy lived, he would always be a patient suffering from the attacks of hysteria.

"When the doctors showed their helplessness, we turned to nature. According to the opinion of one naturopath, the rootcause of my son's ailments was 'overnutrition'. Following his advice, we reduced the amount of food to be given to him. He was now fed with fruits and raw vegetables. At the end of ten months we found that our son had gained two pounds in weight, though his physical condition remained nearly the same. He was not able to walk so far.

"Unsatisfied with the treatment, we decided to consult another naturopath. We consulted an expert naturopath of California who started with fruit and vegetable-juices, carrot-juice being the principal juice. My son was allowed to take honey for sustaining energy. This treatment proved congenial to my son. During the next six months he made a brisk progress. His intestines began to function. He was now able to naturally evacuate his bowels. Mucous and blood disappeared from his faeces.

"By the time my son was 4½ years old, his weight had increased to 39 lbs. His muscular activity was now well developed. He started jumping, running and playing with other children. He used to enjoy a sound sleep at night. The doctor of the hospital to which my son was first admitted in the beginning of his ailments refused to believe him to be the same boy.

"Today my son is twenty-two years old, perfectly healthy

with youthful energy. He has never fallen ill since he started taking carrot-juice. At present also he is devoted to carrot-juice and drinks it joyfully."

(2)

A number of cases have come to light and are still being brought to notice that fatal cancer has been cured with the help of carrot-juice. One exciting instance of the child of a newly married couple is worth quoting.

The first child of this couple was a girl. She was born in 1951. At birth she was apparently beautiful and healthy. But only after a few days her trouble started. When she was two months old, she turned very pale. Her parents consulted their physician. The result of her blood test gave a terrible shock to her parents. The baby girl was a victim of leukaemia. She was immediately shifted to a hospital. She was given twenty-five blood transfusions within five days, but all the efforts to save her life were fruitless and the little girl died at the age of three months.

Their second child, a boy was born in 1953. An examination report of his blood revealed the terrifying fact that the boy also was born with leukaemia. For the parents this was a bolt from the blue. They feared that their dream of a happy and prosperous life would be shattered. During those moments of disappointment and frustration they fortunately came in contact with angel-like Mrs Catherine Ferraro, who had recovered from splenic leukaemia by taking large quantities of carrot-juice daily. Relying on the experience of this woman, they began to give the child 500 ml of carrot-juice daily. For three months the child had been given nothing but carrot juice. After three months, however, other fruits and vegetables were added to his diet. Now the boy was progressing normally and his health was prevented from being worsening. It was proved that the treatment was successful. At the end of one year it was found that his blood count was normal and there were no malignant cells found in blood. Thus, the carrot-juice had evidently performed a miracle in restoring the child's diseased blood stream to a normal healthy condition.

The third child, a baby girl, was born to them in 1954. Blood tests performed at the time of birth showed no evidence of any abnormality. Her blood was free from malignant cells. This was probably due to the fact that the mother had taken carrot-juice regularly throughout her pregnancy. This child was also given absolute carrot-juice diet for three months after birth.

She and her elder brother still continue to take two glasses of carrot-juice each day. Both of them have maintained their good health. The regular intake of carrot-juice has given them protection against other minor and major ailments. There is no wonder that the substance which can cure cancer or prevent cancer can also prove beneficial in other diseases.

***

7. COCONUT

"Coconut water is indispensable in cholera."
— *The School of Tropical Medicine*

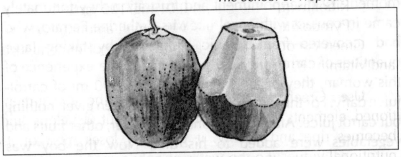

Introduction : The early home of coconut is supposed to be the islands of the Indian and Pacific Oceans. It is now cultivated in almost all the parts of the world.

Qualities : Water of green coconut is cool, exhilarant, nutritious and diuretic. It moderates the colour of urine and quenches thirst. When coconut is not ripe and the formation of the inner kernel has not taken place, its water is less sweet, sour or to some extent astringent. Its water becomes sweet as soon as the formation of the inner kernel takes place. Sugar contained in its water is quickly absorbed. It is safe because it is naturally sterilised and hence free from bacteria.

Analysis of Contents

Water	95.5%
Sodium	105 mg/100 gm
Potassium	312 mg/100 gm
Calcium	29 mg/100 gm
Magnesium	30 mg/100 gm
Iron	0.1 mg/100 gm
Copper	0.04 mg/100 gm
Phosphorus	37 mg/100 gm
Sulphur	24 mg/100 gm
Chlorine	183 mg/100 gm
Vitamin 'B' complex[1]	
Niacin	0.64 mg/100 gm
Pantothenic acid	0.52 mg/100 gm
Biotin	0.02 mg/100 gm
Riboflavin	0.01 mg/100 gm
Pyrodoxin	Very small amount/100 gm

Green coconut water is a good source of mineral salts and vitamin 'B' complex.[2]

Use : Green coconut water contains the above-mentioned elements and vitamins. As the nut develops and becomes ripe and yellow, it gradually loses most of its nutritional virtues. So the water of only a green and tender

1. Food Science, p. 66, March, 1958
2. Council of Scientific Industrial Research – The Wealth of India, Vol. II, p. 278, Delhi

coconut should always be insisted upon for a drink. Fresh water of green coconut should be used immediately. Vitamin 'C' deficiency in coconut water can be met by adding a few drops of lemon juice to it.

Benefits : As green coconut water is diuretic, it is efficacious in urine troubles and kidney-stone.

It is very useful in cholera. On account of vomiting and diarrhoea in cholera, the body gets dehydrated sometimes and loses valuable minerals. This is sometimes fatal. In such circumstances coconut water provides necessary moisture and salts to the body.

As coconut water is antibacterial, it extirpates the cholera germs from the intestines.

Scientists from the school of tropical medicine believe that coconut water rich in natural potassium is superior to injectable potassium salts while treating cholera and its complications.

Vitamin 'B' complex contained in coconut water strengthens the heart and vitalizes the nerves and the digestive system.

***

8. CUCUMBER

"According to recent researches cucumber-juice is a valuable part of the treatment of rheumatic conditions."

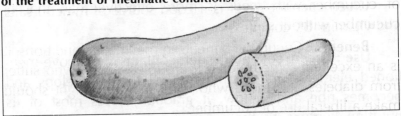

Introduction : Cucumber grows on a vine and it is usually eaten when it is tender. It has two varieties – small and large. It is an oval-shaped vegetable and very delicious to eat.

Qualities : Cucumber is cool, sweet, relishing, light, diuretic, digestive, stimulant of gastric fire and constipating. Dhanvantri Nighantukara says, 'Cucumber allays bile and has a soothing effect. It cures diseases related to urine. It allays burning and checks fainting.' As per latest researches cucumber has a property that gives relief in arthritis. And therefore it is regarded as an important vegetable.

Analysis of Contents

Water	96.4%
Protein	0.4%
Fat	0.1%
Carbohydrates	2.8%
Minerals	0.3%
Calcium	0.01%
Phosphorus	0.03%
Iron	1.5 mg/100 gm
Vitamin 'B'	90 I. U./100 gm

Use : Usually cucumber is cut into pieces before it is eaten. But cucumber-juice possesses many medicinal properties. Juice can easily be extracted from grated cucumber. A juicer is convenient when a large amount of juice is required. A glass of cucumber juice taken on an empty stomach is good for health. As cucumber is very low in calories, it is used in the experiment of reducing obesity. Juice of cucumber with seeds is more effective than that of cucumber without seeds.

Benefits : Cucumber benefits in rheumatic conditions. It is an excellent remedy for uric troubles. Those who suffer from diabetes and those who want to lose weight should make a liberal use of cucumber.

***

9. EMBLICA MYROBALAN
OR
INDIAN GOOSEBERRY (AMLA)

"Vitamin 'C', which Indian gooseberry (*amla*) contains in a large amount, increases the resistance power of the body against disease."

—*Dr. K. V. Giri*

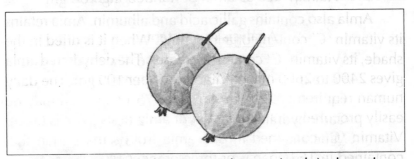

Introduction : Indian gooseberry (amla) has been offering a definite contribution to health ever since man was born. This fruit is abundantly available in winter. No other fruit can stand in comparison with amla as a source of medicinal properties. It is profusely used in the process of complete rejuvenation of the body (Kayakalpa). The chief ingredient of world-famous 'Chyavanprashavaleh' is amla. The amla fruit is as big as a lemon. It is pale-green in colour. It has vertical lines on its outer rind.

Qualities : The taste of amla is somewhat acidic and to some extent acrid. It is delicious and astringent. It vitalizes hair and increases semen. It improves eye-sight and purifies blood. It eliminates all the three 'doshas' namely windiness, bile and cough. Amla is regarded as regimen for man in all seasons without discrimination of nature, time, place or age. Of all fruits Amla is the largest source of vitamin 'C'. It increases the body's resistance against disease.

Analysis of Contents

Water	81.2%
Protein	0.5%

Fat	0.1%
Carbohydrates	14.1%
Fibrous elements	3.4%
Calcium	0.05%
Phosphorus	0.02%
Iron	1.02 mg/100 gm
Vitamin 'C'	600 mg/100 gm

Amla also contains gallic acid and albumin. Amla retains its vitamin 'C' content for a long time. When it is dried in the shade, its vitamin 'C' content increases. The dehydrated amla gives 2400 to 2600 mg. of Vitamin 'C' per 100 gm. The daily human requirement of Vitamin 'C' is 75 mg, which may be easily procured if a little powder of amla or its juice is taken. Vitamin 'C' contained in one amla fruit is more than that contained in 16 bananas or three oranges.

Use : To take the most possible advantages of the valuable ingredients of amla, one should drink its juice. Juice of amla can be obtained by the help of a juicer after discarding the seed from the fruit and cutting the fruit into small pieces. Amla-juice can be obtained also by minutely shredding it and squeezing the pulp through a clean piece of cloth. It can also be obtained by crushing and pounding the fruit in a stone-basin. For cutting amla into pieces a stainless steel knife should be used instead of an iron one. The quality of amla is deteriorated when it comes in contact with iron.

Amla-juice, if taken in the morning on an empty stomach, bestows many benefits.

As the taste of amla is acrid one cannot eat it in sufficient quantity. Therefore, amla-juice is preferable for meeting the necessary requirement. Amla-juice cleanses the mouth and restores taste. If one wishes, a small amount of honey or jaggery may be added to amla-juice for making it palatable. Taking amla-juice is more beneficial than eating its marmalade or any other form of it.

Benefits : Amla-juice is very useful in uric troubles. Drinking fresh amla-juice for two to three months is helpful in conditions of sterility and semen-weakness. Amla-juice is the sure remedy for the eye-weakness and deafness. It is very helpful in constipation, blood impurities, dyspepsia, jaundice, etc. It gives relief also in the weakness of the nerves and the heart.

***

10. FIG

"Small children and pregnant women should invariably eat figs."

—*Dr. Kularanjan Mukerji*

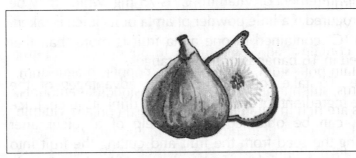

Introduction : The fig has been known to man since the dawn of history. It holds a high place in world commerce. There are many references to the fig in the Bible. It is widely used in Greece, southern Europe, Algeria, Italy and other Mediterranean countries. In Algeria, the average family consumes about 750 kg. of figs every year. In India it is cultivated in Kashmir, Uttar Pradesh, Maharashtra, Karnataka and Gujarat. The fig-tree yields fruits twice a year : in the monsoon and in summer. The summer figs are superior in quality. Ripe fresh figs are delicious and rich in juice.

Qualities : Fresh figs are very nutritious. Figs relieve constipation. Iron contained in the figs is easily digestible and so it is completely assimilated in the body. Figs are cool, delicious and heavy. They check derangement of the bile and

FIG　　　　　　　77

windiness. They eliminate the impurities from blood. In their matured state, they are sweet, soothing and laxative.

Analysis of Contents

Water	80.8%
Protein	3.5%
Fat	0.2%
Carbohydrates	18.7%
Fibres	2.3%
Minerals	0.7%
Calcium	0.06%
Phosphorus	0.03%
Iron	1.2 mg/100 gm
Vitamin 'A'	270 I. U./100 gm

Figs contain plenty of sodium. In addition to sodium, they contain potassium, calcium, iron, copper, magnesium, phosphorus, sulphur and chlorine in considerable amounts. Fresh figs are rich in vitamin 'A'. They also contain vitamin 'B' and 'C' in a moderate proportion. In comparison to fresh fig, dried fig contains three to four times more sugar and minerals when taken weight for weight. The sugar found in the fig is dextrose and fruit sugar. The amount of dextrose in some varieties of fig is about 60 per cent.[1]

Use : Figs can be taken in their juice-form or can be taken by masticating them. If fresh figs are not available, dry figs can be used with the same benefits. Dry figs, if soaked in water for twelve hours, become smooth and soft. Soaking activates the figs' enzymes. A small quantity of juice can be extracted from such soaked figs. The water in which dry figs are soaked should not be discarded. It can be added to thick juice to make it dilute.

Benefits : The juice of fresh figs is diuretic. It therefore alleviates uric troubles. It keeps the liver, the stomach and the

1. Heber W. Youngken – Text-book of Pharmacognosy, p. 282, Toranto

intestines efficient. It removes constipation, fatigue and weakness. It gives relief particularly in a fit of coughing. Small children and pregnant women gain vigour by the use of figs.

***

11. FRENCH BEANS

French beans have a wonderful, balanced combination of natural nutrients. Their juice stimulates the production of insulin. So French beans are useful in diabetes.

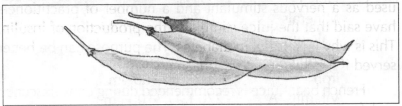

Introduction : The original home of French beans is America. The pods have been used as green vegetables since ancient times. French beans are a winter crop. Their pods generally grow from four to five inches in length.

Qualities : According to the Ayurveda, French beans are heavy, oily, cool, refreshing and antibilious.

Analysis of Contents

Water	82.00%
Protein	1.7%
Fat	0.1%
Carbohydrates	4.5%
Fibre	1.8%
Calcium	0.05%
Phosphorus	0.03%
Iron	1.7 mg./100 gm
Vitamin 'A'	221 I. U./100 gm
Vitamin 'B$_1$'	78 mg/100 gm
Vitamin 'B$_2$'	59 mg/100 gm
Niacin	0.3 mg/100 gm
Vitamin 'C'	14 mg/100 gm

Use : Juice should be extracted by pounding French beans or by grating them and squeezing the grates in a piece of thick cloth. Fresh juice of French beans has a well-balanced combination of nutrients. Though the fresh juice of French beans is not very rich in any particular nutrient, a well-balanced combination of many nutrients in it draws our attention.

Benefits : Therapeutically the juice of French beans is used as a nervous stimulant and a number of practitioners have said that the juice stimulates the production of insulin. This is why it is useful in diabetes. The purpose can be better served if it is taken with cabbage juice.

French bean-juice is recommended during convalescence and for gout. About 150 ml of juice a day is considered sufficient dose for that purpose. In diabetes, the usual requirement is about 275 ml a day.

***

12. GARLIC

"Garlic is the poor man's musk and an indigenous medicine."

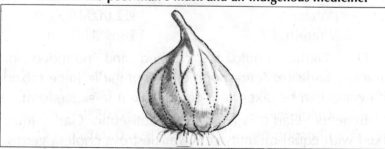

Introduction : The early home of garlic is Middle Asia. It has been very popular in India since ancient times. In Sanskrit, garlic is called 'rasona' which means lacking in only one 'rasa' (taste). There are six 'rasas' (tastes) in all – sweet, sour, saltish, bitter, pungent and astringent. Garlic contains all these 'rasas' (tastes) except sour. Garlic is widely used both as a food and medicine. The root of garlic contains several small cloves forming a compound bulb. Garlic with a single clove is also available and is thought to be more effective than an ordinary garlic bulb. People recognize it by its pungent and offensive smell.

Qualities : Garlic is pungent, warm, heavy, aphrodisiac, oily, delicious, medicinal, digestive and refreshing. It improves the voice and eye-sight. It bestows strength. It is laxative. It kindles gastric fire and is a tonic to hair. It helps the process of calcification in fracture and also is useful in dyspepsia, cough, windiness, worms, heart-disease, oedema, hiccough, asthma, leucoderma, acidity, piles, hard-breathing, colitis, chronic fever, loss of appetite, catarhh, constipation and tuberculosis.

Analysis of Contents

Water	62.8%
Protein	6.3%
Fat	0.1%
Carbohydrates	29.0%
Calcium	0.03%
Phosphorus	0.31%
Iron	1.3 mg/100 gm
Vitamin 'C'	13 mg/100 gm

Use : Garlic should be crushed and pounded for extracting its juice. A teaspoon or two of garlic juice mixed with water can be taken or it can be taken in sauce form.

Benefits : Garlic is a powerful antiseptic. Garlic juice mixed with equal quantity of water destroys cholera germs. Garlic kills both gram positive and gram negative bacteria.[1]

Dr. Minchin pointed out that garlic is a preventive for typhoid. The essential oil sulphide found in the garlic is

1. Morris B. Jacobs, Ph. D.—The Chemistry and Technology of Food and Food Products, p. 1213, Interscience Publishers Inc., New York

an excellent remedy for respiratory diseases. Eminent doctor F. W. Crossman is of the opinion that garlic is a marvellous remedy in the treatment of pneumonia. He used it for several years and, on a paper on this disease, he has written that temperature, respiratory and pulse disturbances—the symptoms of pneumonia—are brought under control (to normal state) within two days only with the use of garlic.

Garlic is a sure remedy in the cases of windiness of any kind. It cures paralysis, stiffness of the whole body, heart-trouble, stomachache and many other ailments.

Garlic has been proved effective as an expectorant and in bronchitis.[1] A number of medical men recommend the use of garlic even in tuberculosis. Garlic dislodges phlegm, induces sleep, improves digestion and helps to gain weight.

Garlic prevents intestinal infection and vitalizes the intestines. It is an excellent medicine for indigestion, dyspepsia, slow flow of digestive juices and gas. Work by Dr. Weiss of Chicago demonstrated the great benefit received in a controlled trial on sufferers from long-standing intestinal disorders such as persistent diarrhoea.

In wounds and ulcerations, garlic is used for counteracting putrefaction. Garlic-juice is employed, together with water, for cleansing infected wounds. When they are thus washed, the condition of the foul ulcer improves within one or two days, the pain ceases and formation of pus decreases. It is necessary to employ the juice diluted with three parts of water. In Russia, it is commonly used for dressing wounds and ulcers.[2]

In the Medical College of Lucknow, 15% garlic juice was applied in dressing to 335 patients suffering from various

1. Sir George Watt, M. B. —Dictionary of Economic Products of India, p. 173, Govt. Press, Calcutta

2. Santi Prakas Gupta and others—Journal of Medical Association, Oct. 1952

types of ulcer for experimental purposes. In one or two days 60 per cent of the patients improved considerably and were discharged from the hospital. The experiment was carried out with a grant from the U. P. Government. When there was excessive pus and slough, it was found necessary to use 50 per cent garlic juice. Garlic is also useful in gout and stones of the kidney and gall bladder.

Garlic has properties to reduce high blood pressure and hence its importance and popularity in the present times has increased by leaps and bounds. It reduces athero-sclerosis and gives relief to the heart. The heart thus becomes vitalized. In the case of ear-pain and deafness a drop of its juice in the ear is beneficial.

*　*　*

13. GINGER

"The perennial use of ginger-juice before meals prevents malignancy of tongue and throat."

— *Rajvaidya Rasiklal Parikh*

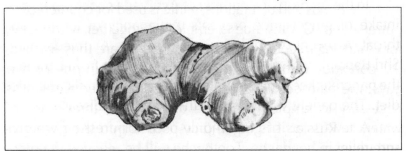

Introduction and Qualities : In Sanskrit, ginger is called 'Vishvaushadha'. It is antirheumatic, stimulant, digestive, laxative, good for eyes and throat and nutritious. Its purgative property destroys intestinal worms which are then eradicated through faeces. Ginger is a good tonic for the intestines. Compared to other poisonous drugs, ginger juice is safe and free from ill-effects.

Analysis of Contents

Water	80.9%
Protein	2.3%
Fat	0.9%
Carbohydrates	12.3%
Iron	2.6 mg/100 gm.

In addition to above nutrients ginger contains vitamin 'A', vitamin 'C', calcium, phosphorus, etc. in small quantities.

Use : Three or four teaspoonfuls of ginger-juice mixed with a very small quantity of mineral salt and a few drops of lemon juice taken half an hour before meals works as an excellent appetiser. Ginger-juice stimulates the secretion of digestive juices. This helps digestion and prevents gas trouble.

Benefits : Juice or small pieces of ginger taken before meals eliminate gas. It dislodges cough and exterminates cattarrh and cold. It corrects cardiac disorders and allays all the abdominal disorders. Ginger-juice is also helpful in oedema, uric troubles, jaundice, piles, asthma, cough, dropsy and other diseases.

In the opinion of a number of Ayurveda experts, a regular intake of ginger-juice prevents malignancy of tongue and throat. A recent example is worth quoting. Ayurvedacharya Shri Bapalal Vaidya treated a patient suffering from cancer of the pancreas keeping him only on ginger juice, milk and juice diet. The patient was cured of the malignant disease.

A few drops of ginger-juice poured into the nose give sure relief in headache. Toothache will be relieved if a piece of ginger is rubbed on the ailing tooth. Ginger also gives relief in cattarrh and sinusitis.

***

14. GRAPES

"The grape is the noblest of all fruits."

— Maharshi Charaka

"Grapes have preventive properties against cancer."

— Dr. J. B. Lust

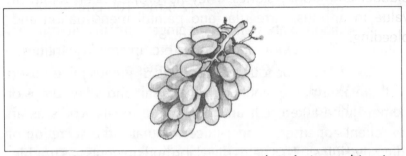

Introduction : In comparison to other fruits, cultivation and growth of grapes is in much more quantity. It is very delicious in taste. One feels like putting a bunch into the mouth, as soon as they are spotted. It is available in large quantities from January to March. Grapes grow on vines. These vines creep on and along pre-made bowers. Grapes are of green, black and violet colours. There are different shapes and sizes of grapes. Grapes of small size are seedless, whereas those of large size have seeds.

Excellent varieties of the grape are cultivated in Europe; in France, and Italy, and in California in America.

Qualities : Maharshi Charaka states that grapes are regimen, sweet, stimulative, soothing, beneficial to the throat, hair, skin and eyes and act as an appetiser. Ripe grapes are oily, diuretic, aphrodisiac, cool and refreshing. They are helpful in eliminating thirst, burning sensation, fever, asthma, leprosy, tuberculosis, irregular menstruation, voice trouble, vomiting, obesity, oedema, chronic jaundice (hepatitis) and other disorders. They decrease gastric acidity.

Sushrut, the great Ayurvedacharya, is of the opinion that grapes help in retaining youth and prevents old age. He states

that grapes are nutritive and a preventive for wasting diseases
(Sushrutasamhita, Ch. 46). They soothe the burning sensation
in the stomach. As they help digestion, gas-trouble is
eliminated.

Grapes give relief in uric troubles, burning sensation in
bladder and kidney-stones. They have often been found of
value in arthritis, irregular and painful menstruation and
bleeding.

Analysis of Contents

Water	85.5%
Protein	0.8%
Fat	7.1%
Carbohydrates	10.2%
Calcium	0.03%
Phosphorus	0.02%
Iron	0.04 mg/100 gm.
Vitamin 'A'	15 I. U./100 gm.
Vitamin 'B$_2$'	10 mg/100 gm.
Niacin	0.3 mg/100 gm.
Vitamin 'C'	10 mg/100 gm.

Raw grapes contain lots of acid elements and less of
sugar but on ripening the amount of sugar increases considerably. The sugar contained in grapes is formed almost by
glucose. The proportion of glucose in grapes is much more in
comparison to other fruits in equal weight. In some varieties of
grapes the sugar content is as high as 50%.[1] The glucose in
grapes is a predigested sugar and is easily absorbed in the body.

Though the iron in grapes is rather scanty, but it is easily
assimilable and hence it is very useful in anaemia. A number
of investigators have found that only 300 ml of grape-juice
can successfully combat progress of anaemia.

1. Henry Sherman, Ph. D.-Chemistry of Food and Nutrition, p. 11, The Macmillan
Company, New York.

Malic, citric and tartaric acids contained in grapes purify blood and stimulate the activity of the bowels as well as the kidneys. Vagbhat, the great Ayurveda expert, had also supported these findings. (Vagbhat Sutrasthana 6 –106)

Use : Though grapes can be taken in their natural form, pure grape-juice has a greater medicinal value. Sufficient amount of grapes can be taken only in the juice form.

Benefits : Grapes, if taken daily, are very good for relieving constipation. They give relief in piles. They have a soothing effect on excessive secretion of bile and the burning sensation in stomach.

Grape-juice brings good results to the patients suffering from general weakness, debility, stagnated weight, dryness of skin, dimness of sight and burning sensation in the body.

Taking grape-juice for a few days removes undesirable heat from the body as the blood is cleansed and cooled.

It has been reported by Dr. J. H. Kellogg, the eminent physician, that a group of soldiers suffering from chronic dysentery stationed themselves for a few days near a grape plantation. The soldiers drank grape-juice and were cured of all symptoms of dysentery.

GRAPES CURE CANCER

A number of experiments conducted in America to detect any anti-cancer properties of grapes have yielded better than expected results.

Here is an amazing example of Mrs. Johanna Brandt who conquered cancer with the grape-fruit diet. This is a living evidence which proves that even women have firm determination and strong will.

At her young age, Mrs. Johanna Brandt suddenly developed severe abdominal pain. In the beginning she resorted to domestic remedies and later to modern medicines. But there was no improvement. She was taken to the hospital for further tests. At the end of all different types of tests, the doctors diagnosed the disease as cancer. Johanna and all the members of her family were struck with grief and fear. The doctors advised Johanna to undergo an operation. But Johanna had formerly met the persons in whom the cancer had worsened after the operation. She was also well aware of the futility of the treatment of cancer by medicines and radiotherapy. So she firmly refused to undergo the customary treatment.

Johanna had come across a book 'Fasting Cure' by Dr. Upton Sinclair. This book inspired her to follow nature-cure. She did multiple short fasts at home. She took food at intervals and resumed fasting. The battle for life lasted for nine years. During every fast tumour stopped growing but did not totally disappear. After nine years, again an X-ray was taken. It showed that the tumour had been divided into two parts. Doctors advised her to immediately undergo an operation. But Johanna Brandt refused again. She continued fasting. Fasting could check the growth of the tumour but the unbearable abdominal pain continued. Three more years passed in this way.

Afterwards purely for the sake of an experiment she began to take grapes alone. This diet proved miraculous. The abdominal pain vanished within a week. Johanna got rid of her cancer just within six weeks. Now there was no trace of tumour in X-ray report. The doctors just could not believe what they saw. After that Mrs. Brandt successfully carried out this grape-juice experiment on a number of patients.

On the basis of her experience Mrs. Johanna has written an interesting book 'The Grape Cure'. The book has been received warmly by laymen and critics alike and has run into many editions.

***

THE GRAPE-CURE

Below is reproduced the method of the grape cure, as stated by Mrs. Johanna Brandt, Dr. Benedict Lust and other experts.

If the disease through biopsy or symptoms is diagnosed as cancer, the patient at first should get his body cleansed through nature-cure treatment. For that he should undertake a two to three days' fast. He should drink plenty of water. If he suffers from constipation enema should be used. A glass or two of cold water should be drunk in the early morning on the day the grape treatment starts. Then half an hour later grape-juice should be taken. The first intake of grape-juice should be at eight o'clock in the morning. Grape-juice should be taken every two hours six or seven times during the day till eight in the evening. 50 to 100 ml of grape-juice should be taken each time. The quantity of the next intake should be gradually increased such that during the whole day 5 to 6 litres of grape-juice is taken by the time of completion of one week. This experiment should be continued for a week or two. If the experiment is found conducive, it should be prolonged for one to two months. As grapes do not provide all the necessary nutritious elements to the body, it is not advisable to continue grape-juice treatment for a very long time.

In the second stage, other fruits should be added to the diet of grape-juice for one to two months. In the third stage, in addition to juices, fruits, vegetables, sprouted grains, sprouted pulses and other such raw food should be taken. One undergoing the grape-cure should not take cooked food for six months. After six months, the fourth stage of this experiment commences. In this stage, a limited quantity of cooked food, according to the individual capacity to digest, should be taken with grapes, salad and other fruits.

Complete rest is essential during the period of grape-juice treatment. The patient should not worry about the debility experienced during this period. This is going to be a very useful experiment. Many reactions take place during this treatment for which the patient should have been mentally prepared. The patient may suffer from diarrhoea. In such a case, the quantity of grape-juice should be reduced or a fasting for a day or two should be observed. When diarrhoea is cured, the intake of grape-juice should be resumed. If the patient suffers from cattarrh, slightly warm grape-juice should be taken.

It is recommended that one who wants to undertake grape-juice therapy should first of all read the inspiring and instructive book 'The Grape-Cure' by Johanna Brandt. It is advisable that one should undergo the treatment under the advice or care of an experienced naturopath. In the Nature Cure Centre of Urulikanchan near Pune, the grape-cure experiments have been successfully performed on thousands of patients. For further information, one should contact the Director of the centre.

* * *

15. GUAVA

"Guava contains much more vitamin 'C' than any other fruit except the Indian gooseberry (*Amla*)".

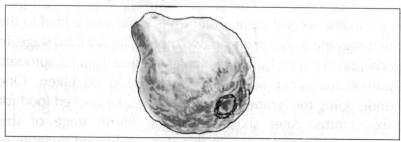

Introduction : The guava tree is indigenous to south America. Today it is widely visible throughout the world. It has been a favourite fruit in India also since ancient times. It is freely available in winter. The guava has two principal varieties : one of them has a white kernel and in the other the kernel is red or pink. The guava with white kernel is sweeter than that with pink kernel. The guava of Prayag and Varanasi in Uttar Pradesh are of excellent quality.

Qualities : Guava is palatable, astringent and sweet. It promotes semen. It is beneficial in constipation. It is cool and it checks the excess flow of bile. It works as an appetiser. It gives relief in burning sensation. It cures delusion and hysteria, and quenches thirst. It destroys intestinal worms. It also gives relief in insanity. It eliminates constipation.

Analysis of Contents

Water	76.1%
Protein	1.5%
Fat	0.2%
Carbohydrates	14.5%
Calcium	0.01%
Phosphorus	0.04%
Iron	1 mg/100 gm
Vitamin 'C'	300 mg/100 gm

Guava contains much more vitamin 'C' than any other fruit except the Indian gooseberry (Amla). When the fruit is over-ripe and soft, its vitamin 'C' potency decreases. The rind of the guava and the kernel nearest to the rind contain the highest amount of vitamin 'C'.[1]

Use : Guava can be eaten directly by masticating it well; but to obtain more nutrients, its juice should be taken. Every 100 ml of the juice contains 70 to 170 milligrams of vitamin 'C'.

Benefits : Guava is beneficial in constipation, blood-impurities, leprosy and other diseases.

* * *

---

1. Carey D. Miller and Katherine Bazore-Fruits of Hawaii, p. 39, University of Hawaii

16. JAMBUL

"In liver diseases jambul-juice works like liver extract."

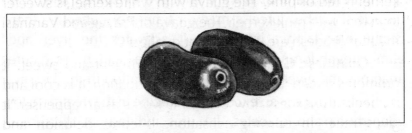

Introduction : Jambul is one of the noblest fruits. Jambul is as valuable in the rainy season as mango is in summer. The jambul fruit is known to all of us. It is delicious, a bit sour and to some extent astringent in taste.

Qualities : According to the Ayurveda, jambul is stimulant to gastric fire, diuretic and constipating. It checks bile and soothes burning sensation.

Analysis of Contents

Water	78.2%
Protein	0.7%
Fat	0.1%
Carbohydrates	19.7%
Calcium	0.02%
Phosphorus	0.01%
Iron	1.00 mg/100 gm

Jambul also contains some amount of vitamin 'C' and vitamin 'B' complex. It also contains folic acid and choline.

Use : Jambul should be soaked in cold water for an hour or two. Then the seed in it should be removed before juice is extracted.

As jambul promotes windiness, it should not be taken on an empty stomach. It should be eaten after meals. Milk should not to be taken three hours before or after the consumption of jambul. Jambul or jambul-juice is forbidden for those who suffer from oedema and vomitting. It is also forbidden for a woman just after delivery and for one who observes fast.

Benefits : Jambul is very effective in spleen and liver disorders. Jambul juice is many a time more effective than costly liver extract injections. It activates the liver and eliminates abdominal pain. It tones up the heart, helps to cure anaemia and gives relief in burning sensation in the kidney.

Jambul juice is an excellent medicine in the treatment for gonorrhoea and diabetes. It cures indigestion, diarrhoea, dysentery, kidney stone and leprosy and removes impurities from the blood.

***

17. LEMON

"My success in climbing Mt. Everest, the highest summit in the world, is greatly due to lemon."

— *Sir Edmund Hillary*

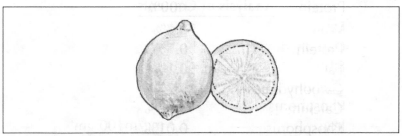

Introduction : In the opinion of Dr. Kularanjan Mukerji, lemon is an orange with more acid and less sugar. The lemon is indigenous to India but is now widely grown all over the world.

Lemon grows in abundance in India, Sri Lanka, Malaysia, Mexico and West Indies. Unripe lemons are green in colour. When they are matured, the colour is changed into yellow. Lemon is a must in the kitchen. It is a universally favourite fruit.

Qualities : The Ayurveda has regarded lemon as a

valuable fruit and admired its properties. Lemon is sour, warm, promoter of gastric fire, light, good for vision, pungent and astringent. It checks the excessive flow of bile and cleanses the mouth. It dislodges phlegm (cough) and expels wind from the digestive tract. It helps in digestion and removes constipation. It prevents vomiting, throat trouble, acidity and rheumatism. It destroys intestinal worms. Though lemon is acidic to the taste, it leaves off alkaline residues in the body. This is why it is useful in all symptoms of acidosis.

Lemon-juice is a powerful antibacterial. It has been proved by experiments and supported by Professor Cox, Dr. J. H. Kellogg, Dr. Wilson and other eminent persons that the bacteria of malaria, cholera, diphtheria, typhoid and other deadly diseases are destroyed in lemon-juice.

Analysis of Contents

Water	85.00%
Protein	1.00%
Fat	0.9%
Carbohydrates	11.1%
Fibres	1.8%
Calcium	0.07%
Phosphorus	0.03%
Iron	2.3 mg/m100 gm
Vitamin 'C'	39 mg/100 gm

It also contains some vitamin 'A'.

Natural vitamin 'C' is much more effective than the synthetic one. vitamin 'C' of lemon-juice is very effective because it is combined with bioflavonoids (vitamin 'P'). In addition to vitamin 'C', lemon also contains niacin and thiamin in small amounts.

Use : One should not take concentrated lemon-juice. It should be diluted with water before taking it. Pure lemon-juice contains acid which is injurious to the enamel of teeth.

The body is well cleansed if lemon-juice mixed with cold water and honey is taken on an empty stomach early in the morning. Warm water may be used occasionally to get relieved of constipation.

Benefits : Lemon-juice prevents or restrains influenza, malaria and cold. Nobel Prize winner, Professor Fanmuller, proved by experiments that lemon is antibacterial. One should take the advantage of these·antibacterial and resistant properties of lemon-juice particularly in the rainy season.

Lemon-juice gives good relief in fever. Lemon-juice mixed with water is useful in quenching the thirst of the patients suffering from diabetes. It gives immediate relief in abdominal disorders. Lemon acts as a sedative for the nerves and the heart and allays troublesome palpitation.

Lemon is especially appreciated for its vitamin 'C' value. When Vasco da Gama made his voyage round the 'Cape of Good Hope' nearly two-thirds of his crew died of scurvy. But at present the recurrence of such a disaster is no longer possible owing to the widespread use of lemon. Innumerable boatmen moving in sea have saved their lives with the use of lemon.

Vitamin 'P' in lemon strengthens the blood vessels and prevents internal haemorrhage. It is, therefore, extremely useful in high blood pressure, in which cerebro-vascular accidents commonly occur.

The most valuable ingredient of lemon, next to vitamin 'C', is citric acid, of which it contains 7.2 per cent.[2]

Lemon contains more potassium than apple or grapes, which is beneficial to the heart.

Lemon is very much useful in maintaining the health of

1. Council of Scientific Industrial Research – The Wealth of India, Vol. II, p. 91, Delhi
2. Henry Edward Cox, Ph. D. – The Chemical Analysis of Foods, p. 122, London

the teeth and the bones. The vitamin 'C' content of lemon helps considerably in calcium metabolism.

Lemon has been used for many years in gout and rheumatism.

Lemon-juice is a diuretic. It, therefore, gives relief in kidney and bladder disorders. It has been used in destroying intestinal worms. It prevents vomiting and helps to cure hepatitis and other innumerable diseases.

Lemon has been proved to be a blessing for mountaineers. In the cases of insufficient oxygen and difficulty in breathing lemon comes to their rescue. Edmund Hillary, the first man to put his foot on the top of Mt. Everest, has admitted that his victory over Mt. Everest was greatly due to lemon.

**

18. MELON

Melon-juice is very beneficial in acute eczema.

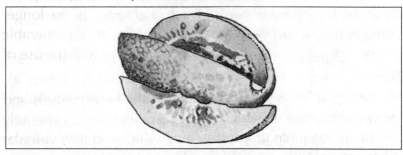

Introduction : Melon is either round or oval in shape. A river-bank with sandy soil is suitable for its growth. Melon with white flesh is known as musk-melon and it is extremely sweet, while melon with green and orange flesh is known as water-melon. It is not as sweet as musk-melon. Both the melons belong to the same genus.

Qualities : Melon is cool and diuretic. It quenches thirst. It gives a welcome cooling and soothing effect during the days of scorching heat.

Analysis of Contents

Water	95.9%
Protein	0.1%
Fat	0.1%
Carbohydrates	3.9%
Calcium	0.11%
Phosphorus	0.01%
Sodium	0.01%
Iron	0.2 mg/100 gm
Vitamin 'A' and 'C'	Trace

As it contains predigested sugar, it provides prompt nourishment.

Use : Melon is mostly composed of water and it contains a little or no fibres. It can, therefore, be taken either directly or in its juice-form.

Benefits : As melon has a cooling property, it soothes burning sensation in the stomach. Its mineral contents eliminate acidity from the body. It also has a property for curing constipation.

Dr. Shircore, once a Civil Surgeon at Murshidabad (Bengal) states : "The pulp of the fruit (melon) is a powerful diuretic and allays kidney diseases. It is also very beneficial in chronic and acute eczema."

As melon-juice promotes cough, one who suffers from asthma or cattarhh and cold should use it discreetly, or use it by making it slightly warm.

***

19. ONIONS

"White onions with about 100 gm of ghee taken early in the morning tone up one's virility. If they are taken for seven days, the body becomes strong. One who takes white onions with ghee regularly rarely falls ill."

—*Aryabhishak*

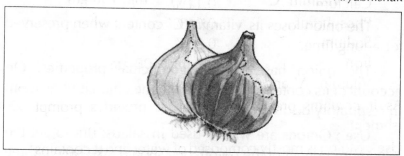

Introduction : The onion has been cultivated since the dawn of human history. Its medicinal properties have been valued in India since ancient times. There are two varieties of onion – white and red.

Qualities : Vigour, lustre of the body and mental power increase with the use of onions.

From medical point of view, white onions are more useful. White onions are stimulant, vitalizing, pungent, promoters of virility, heavy, refreshing, stimulative of gastric fire and lubricous. They produce cough. They increase virility and induce sleep. They are a remedy for tuberculosis, cardiac troubles, dyspepsia, leprosy, piles, swelling and blood impurities.

Analysis of Contents

Water	86.8%
Protein	1.2%
Fat	0.1%
Carbohydrates	11.6%
Calcium	0.18%
Phosphorus	0.05%

Iron	0.7	mg/100 gm
Carotene	50	I. U./100 gm
Vitamin 'B₁'	120	microgram/100 gm
Vitamin 'B₂'	10	microgram/100 gm
Niacin	0.4	microgram/100 gm
Vitamin 'C'	11	mg/100 gm

The onion loses its vitamin 'C' content when preserved for a long time.

The onion has effective germicidal properties. On account of its content of a volatile oil, the onion is very useful in respiratory disorders.

Use : Onions are widely used in salads. But to get the maximum benefit of the onion, one should take two or three teaspoonfuls of onion-juice mixed with honey. White onions should be preferred for medicinal uses.

Benefits : In virile disorders, one should take onion-juice with honey daily in the morning for two to three weeks. This will increase one's virility. The onion saves one from sunstroke. If one suffers from sunstroke, the onion allays it. Eating onion in the morning and at bed-time is beneficial in jaundice.

It is interesting to note that during the plague-epidemic in London, when the contagion spread everywhere, the owners of onion and garlic shops were the only persons who proved immune to the disease.

Two Italian physicians Dr. E. Cuboni and C. Moriondi had used onion-juice to kill T. B. germs. During experiments T. B. germs were injected into the bodies of some guinea-pigs. Thereafter onion-juice was injected into their blood and within short time, it was noticed that T. B. germs were dead. The experiments made by Dr. Heubner have proved that onion-juice is a very effective vermifuge. Unlike many vermifuges, onion-juice is more harmless and free from side-effects.

The onion dislodges mucous and prevents its fresh formation. The onion is beneficial to the aged. The onion is also beneficial in intestinal disorders. The use of onions stimulates the process of peristalsis (contraction and expansion) of the intestines and removes intestinal putrefaction and flatulence. It is also useful in indigestion and biliousness.

The juice of the onion together with sugar is a capital remedy for bleeding piles.

* * *

20. ORANGE

Though it is somewhat acidic to the taste, the orange is an alkali-forming food. After being metabolished in the tissues, it leaves an alkali residue and thus improves the vital resistance of the body.

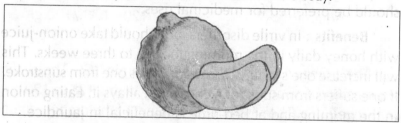

Introduction : Originally a native to Southern China, the orange has now become a favourite fruit all over the world. Its popularity is due to its sourly sweet taste, juiciness, and coolness. There are two seasons for orange cultivation. One is from October to February and the other from March to May. The oranges from Nagpur in Maharashtra are admired. There, oranges grow in abundance.

Qualities : The Ayurveda also has recognised the value of the orange. It works as an appetiser. It cleanses the blood, soothes bile and eliminates windiness. It is cool and refreshing. It cleanses the mouth. It is regimen even in fever. It destroys intestinal worms and allays abdominal pain. It strengthens the bones.

Analysis of Contents

Water	87.8%
Protein	0.9%
Fat	0.3%
Carbohydrates	10.6%
Calcium	0.05%
Phosphorus	0.02%
Iron	0.1 mg/100 gm
Sodium	2.1 mg/100 gm
Potassium	19.7 mg/100 gm
Magnesium	12.9 mg/100 gm
Copper	0.07 mg/100 gm
Sulphur	9.3 mg/100 gm
Chlorine	3.2 mg/100 gm
Vitamin 'A'	350 I. U./100 gm
Vitamin 'B$_1$"	120 I. U./100 gm
Vitamin 'C'	68 I. U/100 gm

The orange is a rich source of vitamin 'C'. The daily requirement of vitamin 'C' is fulfilled by taking 125 to 150 ml of orange-juice. The vitamin 'C' content of the orange is not easily destroyed because it is protected by the citric acid. Besides, vitamin 'C' in the orange is blended with calcium, thereby increasing the qualities of each other. The white membrane, which surrounds the sections of the orange, is an excellent source of calcium.

As orange-juice contains less acid than lemon-juice, it is regarded as superior to the latter. Though the citric acid contained in the orange is somewhat acidic to the taste, it is an alkali-forming food. After being metabolised in the tissues it leaves an alkaline residue and thus improves the vital resistance of the body.[1]

---

1. Henry Sherman – The Science of Nutrition, p. 110. Columbia University Press, New York

Use : The orange is usually taken by masticating it or taken in its juice-form. When there is need for obtaining a large quantity of nutrients, orange-juice is preferred. Those who suffer from cold should add some warm water to orange juice before taking it.

Benefits : To overcome constipation, it is sufficient to take one or two oranges before going to bed and again on rising in the early morning. Oranges are useful in asthma and other bronchial troubles.

During fever, orange-juice greatly helps in supplying necessary nutrition to the patient. It improves digestion and increases appetite. Orange-juice renders the intestinal tract uninhabitable for the hostile microbes and improves the intestinal health.[1] It increases vitality. Orange-juice gives relief to pregnant women who suffer from nausea vomiting.

A cup of orange-juice provides as many calories as three-quarters of milk-cup.[2]

In chronic dyspepsia, food is not well digested. It causes putrefaction in the digestive tract which produces gas. Orange-juice helps in eliminating this putrefaction of food in the stomach. It cleanses the tracts of the stomach and the intestines and thus increases the digestive power of both the digestive organs.

* * *

1. Henry Sherman – Foods, Their Value and Management, p. 72, Columbia University Press, New York

2. J. H. Kellogg, M. D.– The New Dietetics, p. 346, Modern Medicine Publishing Co., Washington

21. PAPAYA

Papaya contains 'papain' which helps to digest food.

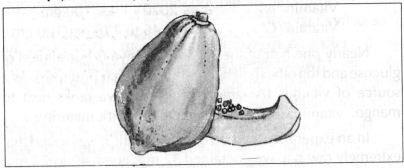

Introduction : The original home of papaya is Mexico and the West Indies Islands, it is believed that, in the early part of the 17th century, it was introduced into India, Africa Australia and other countries.

Papaya is a well-known, cheap and easily available sweet fruit. It grows during the months of February and March as well as May to October. The unripe papaya is green in colour. On its ripening it becomes yellow in colour. The seeds of the ripe papaya are pepper-like black. They are bitter in taste.

Qualities : The ripe papaya is delicious, heavy, warm, oily, laxative and antibilious. It increases virility. It is beneficial to the heart. It helps to alleviate insanity. It is beneficial to the liver. It helps to check splenic enlargement (splenomegaly). It is a good medicine for constipation and urinary disorders.

Analysis of Contents

Water	89.6%
Protein	0.5%
Fat	0.1%
Carbohydrates	9.5%
Minerals	0.4%

Calcium	0.01%
Phosphorus	0.01%
Iron	0.4 mg/100 gm
Vitamin 'A'	2020 I. U./100 gm
Vitamin 'C'	46 to 136 mg/100 gm

Nearly one half of the sugar in papaya is constituted of glucose and the other half by mostly fruit sugar (fructose). As a source of vitamin 'A' among fruits, papaya ranks next to mango. vitamin 'C' in papaya increases with maturity.

In an experiment carried out in Hawaii,[1] it was found that extremely raw papaya contained 32 mg, green 40 to 72 mg, half-ripe 53 to 95 mg and the ripe papaya 68 to 136 mg of vitamin 'C' per 100 gm.

The sugar and vitamin 'C' contents in papaya are highest during the months of May to October. Papaya also contains vitamin 'B$_1$', vitamin 'B$_2$' and niacin.

The white (milky) secretion of raw papaya contains the digestive enzyme papain in significant amount. Papain is a protein-digesting enzyme.

Use : Raw papaya can be used in its juice form. The ripe papaya can be taken in its natural form. Juice can also be extracted from it by adding a little milk or water to it in a mixer. Papaya juice is delicious and refreshing.

Benefits : The raw papaya juice is very helpful in expelling round worms from the digestive tract.[2] The papaya is effective in liver troubles also. It helps to secure proper menstrual flow. The Ayurveda experts have regarded papain as a remedy for abdominal disorders. It is a good medicine for dysentery, hyperacidity, dyspepsia and constipation. It has

---

1. Carey D. Miller, Lucille Louis, Kisako Yanazawa, Honolulu–"Vitamin Values of Food in Hawaii", p. 26, University of Hawaii

2. Dr. R. N. Chopra, M. D., The Medical and Economic Aspects of Some Indian Medical Plants, p. 312, Patna

also been proved useful in anaemia and splenomegaly. In addition to papain, papaya contains enzymes such as arginine (for male fertility), carpain (good for heart) and fibrin (necessary for blood-coagulation).

Dr. Lytton Bernard has claimed rejuvenating properties for papaya for the control of ageing. Papaya cleanses the body completely. To get such cleansing benefits one should take about 200 ml of papaya juice daily. The purpose is rapidly served if one undertakes juice fasting and consumes 200 ml of papaya juice alternated each hour with the equal amount of cucumber juice.

Because of the different types of enzymes contained by papaya, it has been recommended for use as a part of the treatment for cancer. After treatment with antibiotics, the use of papaya juice will hasten the restoration of the friendly symbiotic bacteria in the gut which will have been destroyed by the drugs.

Papaya is also a diuretic. It is therefore beneficial in kidney disorders. The ripe papaya is a sure remedy for constipation. It gives relief in asthma too.

Note : Pimples are removed by rubbing the white pulp of raw papaya on the face. It brings lustre to the face and removes wrinkles.

Some Ayurveda experts believe that papaya causes heat in the body. That is why they advise to avoid papaya in pregnancy, and in fever.

The seeds of the ripe papaya are used for quenching thirst and for destroying intestinal worms.

A poultice of the leaves of a papaya plant is beneficial in neuralgia (nerve-pain) and elephantiasis.[1]

***

1. Council of Scientific Industrial Research – The Wealth of India, Vol. II, p. 79, Delhi

22. PINEAPPLE

"As the pineapple contains sufficient chlorine, it stimulates the activity of the kidneys and helps to remove waste products from the body."

—Sir George Watt

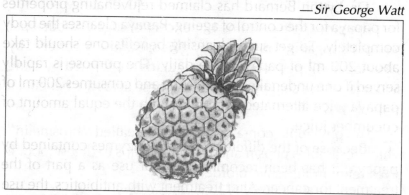

Introduction : The pineapple is believed to be a native of Brazil and was introduced in Europe by Columbus, the famous navigator. Afterwards it spread everywhere. There is a reference that the Portuguese brought it to India in 1502 A. D.

It is freely grown in India. It is easily available during the months of July to November.

The pineapples grown in Burma, Malaysia and the Philippine Islands are considered to be of excellent quality.

Qualities : The Ayurveda has brought to light many of the properties of pineapple. The ripe pineapple is a diuretic. It destroys intestinal worms and soothes bile. It is delicious and digestive. It expels gas. It is beneficial to the heart and effective in abdominal disorders, jaundice and anaemia.

Analysis of Contents

Water	86.5%
Protein	0.6%
Fat	0.1%
Sugar	12.0%
Calcium	0.12%

Phosphorus	0.01%
Iron	0.9 mg/100 gm
Vitamin 'A'	60 I. U./100 gm
Vitamin 'B$_2$'	120 I. U./100 gm
Vitamin 'C	63 mg/100 gm

The pineapple contains 12 per cent of sugar. About 4 per cent of its sugar is constituted by glucose and 7.5 per cent by cane-sugar. 87 per cent of its total acids are formed by citric acid and 13 per cent by malic acid. These acids are beneficial to the body.

The pineapple contains an enzyme called "brosmelin" which resembles pepsin and therefore helps to digest food. It gives relief in digestive diorders.

Use : The pineapple should not be taken on an empty stomach. The upper rind and the innermost flesh of the pineapple should be discarded. The remaining portion should be cut into pieces. Juice should be extracted from these pieces. Raw pineapple or excessively ripe pineapple should be avoided during pregnancy.

Benefits : Fresh pineapple juice exercises a soothing effect on the throat. It is very useful in preventing affections of the vocal organ. In diphtheria it is used for removing the dead membranes from the throat. This antiviral property of the pineapple juice has been confirmed even by the Ayurveda experts.[1] As per their opinion pineapple juice allays bile, destroys intestinal worms and is beneficial to the heart.

Chlorine contained in the pineapple juice stimulates the activity of the kidneys and helps to remove toxic elements and waste products from the body.[2] It also gives relief in cellulitis.

***

1. An Indian Dietarian–Food and Nutrition in India, p. 191, Calcutta
2. W. B. Hays–Fruits Growing in India, p. 221, Allahabad

23. POMEGRANATE

"Pomegranate juice is very easy of digestion and it allays cardiac pain."

—-Dr. Wilson Popenoe, New York

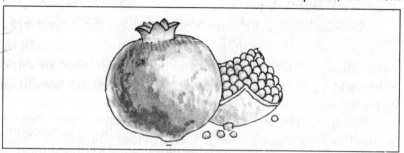

Introduction : Pomegranate is believed to be a native of Persia and Afghanistan. It has been used in India for centuries. In ancient times King Solomon had a garden exclusively of pomegranates. Before a few years Muskati pomegranates were very popular. But, now pomegranates of excellent qualities grow also in India. Pomegranates from Dholka (Gujarat) are very popular. Pomegranate is a summer fruit.

Qualities : Pomegranate has three varieties – sweet, sourly sweet and sourly sweet with astringent taste. Sweet pomegranates are excellent. They are delicious, light, astringent, constipating and lubricous. They increase intellect. They vitalize the body and satisfy hunger. According to Ayurveda, they are 'tridoshnashaka' i.e. they effectively alleviate all the three ailments (windiness, biliousness and cough). They are also beneficial in thirst, burning sensation, fever, cardiac trouble, mouth-disease and vocal disorders. Furthermore, they cure dysentery and increase blood and vitality.

Analysis of Contents

Water	78%
Protein	1.7%
Fat	0.1%
Carbohydrates	14.5%

Calcium	0.01%
Phosphorus	0.07%
Iron	0.03 mg/100 gm
Vitamin 'B$_2$'	10 mg/100 gm
Vitamin 'C'	16 mg/100 gm

Sugar content of pomegranate is in the predigested form and contains only 0.15 per cent of sucrose.

Use : Pomegranate juice is a bit costly; but compared to other juices it is easily digestible. The juice can be extracted by squeezing its seeds in a piece of cloth. Only sweet pomegranates should be selected for medicinal uses. Pomegranate is effective in all types of fevers. It provides nutrition without giving any undue exertion to the digestive system.

Benefits : It is a tonic for the heart and allays cardiac pain.[1] It cures vocal and mouth diseases. It has a soothing effect on the burning sensation in the stomach. It increases appetite and gives relief in anaemia. It is also useful in diarrhoea, dysentery and cough.

***

24. POTATOES

"As the potato is alkaline, it is very helpful in maintaining the alkali reserve of the body and preventing acidosis."

—Dr. J. H. Kellogg, M. D.

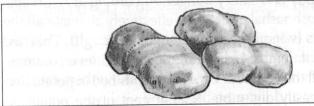

Introduction : The potato is the most popular and widely used vegetable in the world. It is a native of Southern

---

1. Wilson-Popenoe–Manual of Tropical and Sub-tropical Fruits, p. 375, Macmillan & Co., New York

America. The potato was brought to Europe for the first time by Columbus, on his return from the New World, after his second voyage.

In the 16th century, the potato was looked upon as a poisonous tuber. Its food value was realised when in the year 1771 a prize was offered in France for the discovery of an article of food which could be used as substitute for wheat in times of famine. Since then it has become very popular,and its importance as a food article has been recognised.

At present the potato is widely cultivated in India. It grows on a vine in the form of an underground root. Potatoes from Mahabaleshwar in Maharashtra are of excellent quality.

Qualities : Potatoes are cool, delicious, heavy, dry and energising. They increase virility. They cure leprosy but promote cough and gas.

Analysis of Contents

Water	74.7%
Protein	1.6%
Carbohydrates	22.9%
Calcium	0.01%
Phosphorus	0.03%
Iron	0.7 mg/100 gm
Vitamin 'A'	40 I. U./100 gm

The potato is also a source of vitamins 'B_1', 'B_2', niacin and contains vitamin 'C' too. The abovementioned contents indicate that all the virtues of cereals are imbibed in potato. Its nutrients are easily digestible. 95 per cent of the potato is digestible. It is completely absorbed in the body within two and half hours after eating it.

The most important contribution of the potato is its vitamin 'C' content. Scurvy in Europe has become more and more uncommon with the increase in the use of potato.

The amount of vitamin 'C' in potato decreases with the passage of time.

Use : The potato should be cut only when it is to be served otherwise it loses much of its vitamin 'C'. If potato is peeled before it is steamed or boiled, most of its nutrients are destroyed.

In foreign countries raw potato-juice is widely used. It is desirable that this custom comes in vogue in India too. A juicer should be used for extracting juice from potatoes. The other method for getting juice is to crush or pound potatoes and then extract the juice through a cloth. That portion of the potato with green discolouration should be cut and discarded because it contains a toxic substance called 'solanine'. Besides, if the potato is found sprouted, the sprouted portion should be cut and discarded before its use.

Benefits : The potato prevents the fermentative process in the intestine and helps the growth of friendly bacteria in the digestive tract. Potato juice gives good relief to the patients suffering from duodenal and gastric ulcers. It gives relief in constipation and pile. As the potato contains soda and potash, it prevents acidosis, and maintains the alkali reserver of the body.[1] It is useful to the patients suffering from gout, as the mineral elements of the potato help the elimination of uric acid from the body. Potato and potato-juice give encouraging results in several skin-diseases especially in eczema. For this, potato-juice should be drunk as well as applied to the diseased part of the skin.

***

---

1. J. H. Kellogg, M. D.– The New Dietetics, p. 280, Modern Medicine Publishing Co., Washington

25. PUMPKIN

For centuries the Balkan peasants of Russia have used the juice of pumpkin and its seeds to maintain the health of the prostate gland.

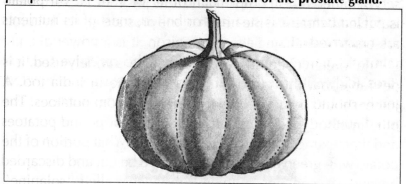

Introduction : There is hardly any fruit which is as big as the pumpkin. With pedicle the pumpkin can be preserved even for a year.

Qualities : The pumpkin preserves and increases virility. It is vitalizing, sweet and vermifuge. It is cool, heavy, dry, laxative, good for the heart and diuretic. It removes kidney disorders and controls the secretion of bile. It is universally regimen.

Analysis of Contents

Water	92.6%
Protein	1.4%
Fat	0.1%
Carbohydrates	5.3%
Minerals	0.6%
Calcium	0.01%
Phosphorus	0.3 %
Iron	0.7 mg/100 gm
Vitamin 'A'	84 I. U./100 gm
Vitamin 'B'	200 I. U./100 gm

No other vegetable or fruit contains as much vitamin 'B' as the pumpkin.

Use : One should use only the ripe (matured) pumpkin and never the raw one. While extracting its juice, its seeds should also be used with the pulp.

Benefits : The pumpkin and the juice of its seeds are useful in maintaining the health of the prostate gland. Its juice possesses neutralizing effect on poison. It is a powerful anti-helmintic or remover of worms from the digestive tract. It cures acidity. Its juice is diuretic. The kidneys are stimulated gently by the juice. It gives relief in swelling, kidney-stone and diabetes.

* * *

26. SWEET LEMON

"The juice of sweet lemon increases vitality and resistance against diseases."
—*Dr. Kularanjan Mukerji*

Introduction : The sweet lemon, one of the most delicious fruits, is known to all. In India the sweet lemon is one of the most popular fruits. It is considered indispensable in illness. The sweet lemon with thin rind possesses valuable nutrients. It belongs to lemon genus.

Qualities : The sweet lemon is sweet, delicious and cool. It quenches thirst. It is refreshing and heavy. It promotes virility. It is somewhat constipating. It is effective in windiness, biliousness, cough, vomiting, dehydration, blood-impurities and dyspepsia. Alkaline elements contained in the sweet lemon reduce acidity of the stomach. Its juice increases vitality and resistance power against diseases.

Analysis of Contents

Water	84.6%
Protein	1.5%
Fat	1.0%
Carbohydrates	10.9%
Calcium	0.09%
Phosphorus	0.02%
Vitamin 'A'	26 I. U./100 gm
Iron	0.3 mg/100 gm
Vitamin 'C'	63 mg/100 gm

Use : Chewing sweet lemon cleanses and strengthens the teeth. Its fibrous elements are useful in removing constipation. However, to get the maximum benefit of its properties, its juice should be taken. Juice can easily be extracted from it with the help of a hand-juicer. Those who are easily affected by cold should warm the juice a bit before taking it or add two spoonfuls of ginger juice.

Benefits : In fever, when any other food is prohibited, sweet lemon-juice proves to be a boon, providing nourishment to the body. Sweet lemon-juice allays acidity and is an excellent appetiser. It rapidly normalizes the impaired digestion.

***

27. TOMATOES

The tomato is an excellent food for diabetics and for those who desire to reduce their weight.

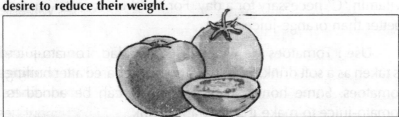

Introduction : The tomato is a native of South America. Sir Walter Raleigh brought it to Europe. It is said that it was introduced into India from Europe.

Qualities : According to the Ayurveda, the tomato is light, lubricous, warm, stimulant, appetiser, laxative and a remover of cough and windiness.

Analysis of Contents

Water	94.3%
Protein	0.9%
Fat	0.4%
Carbohydrates	3.9%
Minerals	0.9%
Vitamin 'A'	100 I. U./100 gm
Vitamin 'C'	39 mg/100 gm

The tomato contains some vitamin 'B_1' and 'B_2'. The minerals contained in the tomato include calcium, phosphorus, sulphur, potassium, magnesium, chlorine, sodium, iron and idodine. It also contains citric, phosphoric and malic acids which purify the blood.

The tomato is rich in vitamin 'A'. Five small tomatoes are sufficient to supply necessary vitamin 'A' for a day. Weight for weight tomatoes contain more vitamin 'A' than butter. It is remarkable that the vitamin 'C' content contained in the tomato is not quickly destroyed because it is protected by the acid it contains. The vitamin 'C' content of the tomato increases as it ripens.[1] Only ripe tomatoes contain vitamin 'B_2'. Only 150 ml of tomato juice supplies one-third of vitamin 'C' necessary for a day. For children, tomato-juice is better than orange-juice.[2]

Use : Tomatoes are widely used as salad. Tomato-juice is taken as a soft drink. Soup can also be prepared after boiling tomatoes. Some honey, date or jaggery can be added to tomato-juice to make it a palatable drink.

---

1. Michael G. Wohl, M. D. –Dietotherapy, p. 947. W. B. Saunders Co., Philadelphia
2. Carleton Ellis, S. B., F. C. S. and Annie Louise Macleod, Ph. D.-Vital Factors of Foods, p. 83, London

Benefits : As the tomato has a very low carbohydrate content, it is a very good food for diabetic patients and for those who want to reduce their body weight.

Tomato-juice cleanses the stomach and the intestines. It is also useful in kidney disorders. It removes indigestion, gas and constipation. It gives relief in liver-diseases. As the iron of the tomato is easily digestible, it is completely absorbed in the body. Hence tomato-juice is very important for anaemic patients. Tomato soup can be given also in fever.

There is a reference that in Guy's Hospital at London, patients suffering from eye-troubles and weakness were cured by tomato-juice. In 'The Cancer Hospital' at New York, the patients are given tomatoes and tomato-juice.

* * *

28. TURMERIC

Turmeric vitalizes the liver by stimulating it. It has the property of purifying the blood.

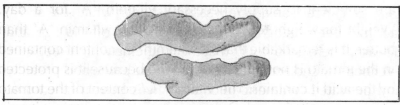

Introduction : Powdered turmeric is freely used while cooking; but green turmeric is rarely used. It is desirable that green turmeric should be widely used. Turmeric grows under the ground in a root-form. It is yellow in colour.

Qualities : According to the Ayurveda, turmeric is bitter, pungent, warm, stimulant, vermifuge, cleanser and the remover of cough, swelling and gas. It is dry in nature. It heels wounds, stimulates the liver, promotes lustre of the body and improves the colour of the skin. It is useful in cold, cough, gas, blood-impurities, leucoderma, diabetes, wounds, skin-diseases, swelling, anaemia, dyspepsia, etc.

Analysis of Contents

Water	13.1%
Protein	6.3%
Fat	5.1%
Carbohydrates	69.4%
Minerals	3.5%
Calcium	0.15%
Phosphorus	0.28%
Iron	18.6 mg/100 gm
Vitamin 'A'	50 I. U./100 gm

Use : Juice can be extracted by pounding turmeric. Two or three teaspoonfuls of turmeric-juice should be taken directly or mixed with water.

Benefits : Turmeric possesses a unique property, not found in any other substance, to stimulate and strengthen the liver. The ancient books of the Ayurveda have accepted this fact. Modern dietarians also have accepted this property of turmeric. In the February 1937 issue of British official medical journal 'Lancet', an article was published in which the above fact had been recognized. Turmeric wards off old age and disease. There is no doubt that the medicine which keeps the liver healthy and activates it can make the entire body healthy and activated. Trumeric-juice also gives benefit in chronic jaundice.

Turmeric-juice is a purifier of the blood and remover of cough. Turmeric juice drops have been found to deliver favourable effect in eye-diseases such as glaucoma, corneal ulcer and conjunctivitis. If fresh turmeric-juice is taken regularly in the morning and at evening, it gives benefit in leucoderma and swellings of legs and arms. Fresh turmeric-juice or turmeric powder mixed with warm milk gives sure benefits in cough and cold. A warm ointment of turmeric-powder can be beneficially applied over sprained and swollen body parts.

Turmeric-juice checks mucous coming out of the nose,

the throat or the wind-pipe. It dries mucous membranes and reduces phlegm.

Turmeric is very beneficial in skin-diseases. It purifies the blood and breast-milk. The skin becomes smooth and fair-complexioned. Skin-diseases are cured when massaged with butter mixed with turmeric.

***

29. WATERMELON

"In scorching summer days, nothing is more soothing than the juice of the watermelon."

—Dr. J. H. Kellogg

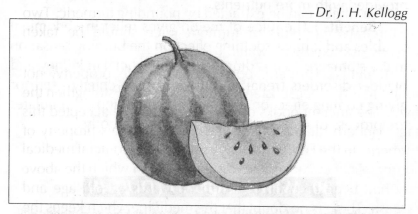

Introduction : The watermelon is indigenous to Africa. It is now a favourite fruit in all the parts of the world. Growing on a vine this fruit is round in shape and weighs generally between 1 to 12 kgs. The pulp (kernel) of the watermelon is reddish in colour and very sweet in taste. The pulp contains black seeds.

Qualities : According to the Ayurveda, the watermelon is cool, diuretic, energising and delicious. It satisfies thirst and hunger, gives nutrition and allays biliousness.

Analysis of Contents

Water	95.7%
Protein	0.1%
Fat	0.2%

Carbohydrates	3.8%
Calcium	0.1%
Phosphorus	0.01%
Iron	0.2 mg/100 gm
Niacin	0.2 mg/100 gm
Vitamin 'B$_1$'	2.0 micogram/100 gm
Vitamin 'E'	1 mg/100 gm

Use : The watermelon can be eaten directly after discarding its thick rind and seeds. Its juice also can be taken. Since the juice can be taken in large quantity, the body is provided with more nutrients.

Benefits : The juice of melon gives relief in abdominal troubles and it has a soothing effect on the burning sensation in the stomach. As it is diuretic, it is beneficial in kidney and bladder disorders (renal dysfunction). It is chiefly used for giving cooling effect on the body and the mind. It stimulates the process of rejuvenation going on in the body.

***

30. WHITE GOURD (DUDHI)

The fresh juice of the white gourd is as nourishing as mother's milk. A bowl made of bitter gourd is used for swimming, while the white gourd enables one to cross the ocean of disease.

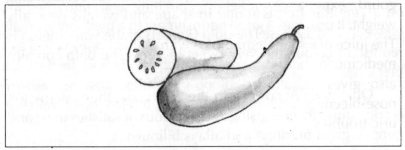

Introduction : Gourd is of two varieties : sweet and bitter. Some are long and some are oval in shape. White gourd is a popular vegetable. It grows on a vine. Sweet gourd is used for eating. Bitter gourd is called a bowl.

Qualities : White gourd is cool, laxative, nutritive and delicious. It promotes virility. It is refreshing and good for the heart. It gives vigour and controls cough and the secretion of bile.

Analysis of Contents

Water	96.3%
Protein	0.2%
Fat	0.1%
Carbohydrates	2.9%
Calcium	0.02%
Phosphorus	0.01%
Iron	0.7 mg/100 gm

As the white gourd has a very low carbohydrates content, it can be used freely by even diabetic patients.

Use : In addition to its use as a vegetable, it can also be used as a drink in its juice-form. In fever the juice of white gourd is very helpful. Juice can be extracted from it with the help of a juicer. It should be noted that only tender, younger, white gourd should be selected for food.

Benefits : A T. B. patient, if given the juice of white gourd, experiences relief in coughing and puts on little weight. It provides a good nourishment to a pregnant woman. The juice of white gourd mixed with a little honey works as a medicine for burning sensation in the body and the throat. It also gives benefits in blood-impurities, abscess, allergy, nose-bleeding and other ailments. It also gives relief in uric troubles.

Boiled white gourd eliminates constipation and reduces blood-acidity.

***

31. GREEN LEAFY VEGETABLES

Some people avoid eating leafy vegetables because they believe that leafy vegetables are one kind of grass. These people lose the benefits of valuable nutrients of leafy vegetables.

Another reason why some people avoid leafy vegetables is that leafy vegetables are believed to be infested with small insects. It is true that some time leafy vegetables do contain small insects, but that fear can be avoided by purchasing them with careful selection. Green leafy vegetables contain chlorophyll. It is a powerful insecticide. Leafy vegetables when chewed prevent decomposition of food particles between the teeth and destroy the germs which cause putrefaction of the teeth. Chlorophyll also destroys hostile bacteria from the intestines and the body. Chlorophyll contains protein of high quality. It satisfies protein requirement to some extent of those who are on juice-diet or on juice-fasting.

The iron content of fresh green leafy vegetables gives relief in anaemia and weakness. Green leafy vegetables are rich in minerals which reduce acidity of the stomach and the body. The constitution of human blood is alkaline. Hence the food that contains minerals is most suitable for man's consumption.

It is not true that the juice or the soup of leafy vegetables is unpalatable. The juice of green vegetables can be made tasty and delicious by their proper combination. The mixture of the juice of leafy vegetables and apple or carrot-juice makes a delicious and refreshing drink.

Those who suffer from peptic or duodenal should not eat leafy vegetables directly because the fibres which leafy vegetables contain might harm them. Juice taken without fibres is not harmful. Those who suffer from diarrhoea or dysentery should restrict the consumption of leafy vegetables. The spinach contains a good amount of oxalates. It should, therefore, be avoided by those who suffer from kidney-stone. They should minimize the consumption of other leafy vegetables also.

Below are described the properties of various leafy vegetables :

CORIANDER

Introduction : We are all well familiar with coriander. It is used in various ways in our daily diet.

Qualities : Coriander is fragrant, appetising, digestive, cool, good for vision, antibilious and agreeable to the heart.

Analysis of Contents

Water	87.9%
Protein	3.3%
Fat	0.6%
Carbohydrates	6.5%
Calcium	0.14%
Phosphorus	0.06%
Iron	10 mg / 100 gm
Vitamin 'A'	10460 to 12600 I. U./100 gm
Vitamin 'C'	135 mg/100 gm

The above list shows that coriander is a rich source of vitamin 'A' and iron.

Use : Coriander is cut into minute shreds and mixed with vegetables and other food items. This gives a special flavour to the food and makes it easily digestible. We usually prefer the paste-like sauce (chutney) of coriander and take it regularly with cereals. But drinking its juice has special advantages.

Benefits : As coriander contains vitamin 'A', it is beneficial to the eyes. A few drops of coriander-juice instilled into the eyes give benefit to them. Coriander-juice is very effective in anaemia.

AMARANTH (TANDALJA/CHAULAI)

Introduction : This leafy vegetable is available throughout the year and is freely used in every house. It is full of excellent nutritious contents and qualities. People relish it. As it enjoys the topmost position among all leafy vegetables, amaranth can be described as the best of all.

Qualities : Amaranth is delicious, cool, appetising, a kindler of gastric fire, diuretic, light, dry, digestible and laxative. It allays biliousness. It purifies blood and eliminates the ill-effects of poison. It dislodges phlegm. It is effective in leprosy and allergy. It gives relief in cough. Its soup is regimen in fever. When digested, it becomes alkaline in nature.

Analysis of Contents

Water	85%
Protein	3%
Fat	0.3%
Carbohydrates	8.1%
Minerals	3.6%
Calcium	0.8%
Phosphorus	0.05%
Iron	22.9 mg/100 gm
Vitamin 'A'	2500 to 11000 I. U./100 gm
Vitamin 'B'	173 I. U./100 gm
Vitamin 'C'	173 mg/100 gm

The iron content which is in abundance in amaranth is very useful in anaemia. Its vitamin 'C' content works effectively in the treatment of leprosy.

Use : It is popularly used as a cooked vegetable. But, for the cure of disease or for getting the maximum benefit of its properties one should consume its raw juice. Juice can be extracted by pounding it.

Benefits : Fresh juice of amaranth is diuretic and hence gives relief in uric troubles. It also gives relief in gynecic disorders.

It helps to eliminate ill-effects of poison or a poisonous drug. Hence if the juice of amaranth is taken frequently, unnecessary and unwanted substances and toxic elements will be eliminated from the body. The vitamin 'A' content of amaranth is useful for the eyes. It cures eye-diseases. Raw juice of amaranth if taken for a few days checks the falling hair, and helps the growth of new hair.

Note : If amaranth is taken by masticating it, it relieves constipation and removes ulcer in the mouth and greasiness of teeth.

BEZIL (TULSI)

Bezil has been recognized as a medicine ever since the dawn of civilization. Its medicinal properties have made it so popular that people regard it with devotion and worship it. Bezil has two varieties : black and white. Black bezil is considered to be superior to white bezil in merit. On account of its multifarious properties, our ancient sages have given it a religious significance so that every Indian·house might have a bezil-plant grown near it. Bezil plant grows only in India. It is part and parcel of Indian life.

Qualities : Bezil is bitter, pungent, warm, fragrant, light, appetising and dry in nature. It cures gas-trouble, cough, swelling, intestinal worms, vomiting, skin-diseases and kidney-disorders. It is good for the heart and the eyes. It expels intestinal worms. It is believed that the bezil-plant emits one kind of gas which purifies the polluted atmosphere around it.

Use : Take two to three spoonfuls of bezil-juice either alone or mixed with some other palatable juice.

Benefits : Two to three spoonfuls of bezil-juice taken on an empty stomach in the morning increases vitality and lustre of the body. It is a good nerve-tonic. It enhances the memory-power.

Bezil-juice kindles gastric fire. It is definitely effective against hyper-acidity, dysentery, colitis and other digestive disorders.

A spoonful of bezil and ginger-juice mixed with honey works as a good medicine for fever, cough and asthma.

Bezil-juice is a specific remedy for malaria. It allays cold, catarrh and headache. It has strengthening effects on the kidneys. It brings down the level of cholesterol in blood.

Two drops of bezil-juice put in the eyes twice a day bring good results in the treatment for night-blindness. Bezil-juice if applied on the body cures allergy. A few drops of bezil-juice are put in the ear to treat any ear-trouble.

A simple decoction prepared by boiling bezil, ginger and green tea leaves in water is very delicious and nourishing one.

SPINACH (PALAKH)

The spinach is the most popular leafy vegetable. It is cultivated on a large scale in almost every part of India. At present, it is the most esteemed green leafy vegetable.

Qualities : Spinach is a bit pungent, sweet, digestible, cool and dry. It stimulates peristalsis and is a mild laxative. It is easy to digest and assimilate. It has a satisfying quality. It is heavy and palatable. It eliminates cough, asthma and toxic elements.

Analysis of Contents

Water	91.7%
Protein	1.9%
Fat	0.9%
Carbohydrates	4.00%
Minerals	1.5%
Calcium	0.06%
Phosphorus	0.01%
Iron	5 mg/100 gm
Vitamin 'A'	2600 to 3500 I. U./100 gm
Vitamin 'B'	70 I. U./100 gm
Vitamin 'C'	48 mg/100 gm

It also contains magnesium, sulphur, sodium, silicon and potassium in minute quantities.

Use : The spinach is an agreeable vegetable. It is often cooked as a green vegetable. Its soup also can be taken by boiling it. But its raw juice gives the maximum benefits of its contents.

Benefits : As the iron of spinach is easy of digestion, it is employed as a food medicine in anaemia with satisfactory results. The minerals which spinach contains reduce acidity and bestow health. Its juice is diuretic. It allays bile-disorders. It is very effective against gynecic diseases.

Note : Spinach contains salts of oxalic acid in good proportion. Hence it is harmful to people likely to get kidney stone-trouble. Therefore, they are advised to make restricted use of spinach.

PARSLEY MINT (PHUDINA)

Introduction : Mint is well-known for its medicinal properties and is used nearly in every house regularly.

Qualities : Mint is palatable, heavy, lubricous, warm, appetising, vermifuge, constipating and good for the heart. It expels gas. It is useful in cough, dyspepsia, dysentery, gastroenteritis and diarrhoea.

Analysis of Contents

Water	83.00%
Protein	4.8%
Fat	0.6%
Carbohydrates	8.00%
Minerals	1.6%
Calcium	0.20%
Phosphorus	0.08%
Iron	15.6 mg/100 gm
Vitamin 'A'	2700 I. U./100 gm

Use : Juice can be extracted by pounding mint.

Benefits : A mixture of two teaspoonfuls of mint-juice, one teaspoonful of lemon-juice and two teaspoonfuls of honey is a powerful medicine for abdominal troubles. Vitamin 'E' content of mint prevents the wear and tear of the body and energizes blood vessels. It is vermifuge. A mixture of equal quantities of mint-juice, onion-juice and lemon-juice makes a specific remedy for cholera. A few drops of mint-juice if put in the nostrils bring good results in catarrh and nose-trouble. Applying mint-juice on ringworm has beneficial effects.

FENUGREEK (METHI)

Introduction : Fenugreek leafy vegetable is one of the most popular leafy vegetables. Because of its recuperative properties it has become a favourite vegetable.

Qualities : Fenugreek leafy vegetable is pungent, bitter and warm. It promotes bile. It is appetising, light and dry. It prevents diarrhoea. It is good for the heart. It expels gas. It gives benefits in dyspepsia, vomiting, cough, rheumatism, piles, intestinal worms and other ailments.

Analysis of Contents

Water	81.8%
Protein	4.9%
Fat	0.9%
Carbohydrates	9.8%
Minerals	1.6%
Calcium	0.47%
Phosphorus	0.05%
Iron	16.9 mg/100 gm
Vitamin 'A'	3900 I. U./100 gm
Vitamin 'B'	70 I. U./100 gm

Use : Fenugreek leafy vegetable should be taken in its juice-form. Juice should be extracted from raw vegetable. It can be taken in its soup-form also. Soup should be prepared from fenugreek boiled or steamed in a pressure-cooker. A juice-mixer is convenient for preparing the soup.

Benefits : Fenugreek is regimen for pregnant women and for patients suffering from fever and dyspepsia. Two spoonfuls of fenugreek-juice removes indigestion. It gives relief in piles. Juice of fenugreek leafy vegetable mixed with black raisins gives relief in bleeding. As fenugreek contains a good amount of iron, it is very effective in anaemia.

RADISH AND ITS LEAVES

Introduction : Like carrot, radish also grows in the form of root under the ground. It has two varieties – white and red. Its plant which grows above the ground consists of radish leaves. Radish is the staple food of the Japanese.

Qualities : Tender radish is saline, bitter, warm, light, appetising, stimulant of gastric fire, digestive, sweet, constipating, pungent, laxative, good for the heart and vitalizing. It cures asthma, cough, piles, eye-diseases, gas-trouble, vocal disorders and other diseases. The arsenic content of radish has a beneficial effect on the thyroid gland. The juice of radish leaves is diuretic. According to the Ayurveda, it promotes digestion and eliminates all the three principal systemic disturbances (windiness, biliousness and cough).

Analysis of Contents

Water	94.4%
Protein	0.7%
Fat	0.1%
Carbohydrates	4.2%
Minerals	0.4%
Calcium	0.05%
Phosphorus	0.03%
Iron	0.04 mg/100 gm
Vitamin 'B'	60 I. U./100 gm

Besides these, radish contains vitamin 'A' and 'C' in small quantities. In minerals, it has potassium, sodium arsenic, magnesium, sulphur, salicylic acid and sodium chloride.

Use : One should take the juice of radish and its leaves.

Benefits : Radish promotes digestive power. It destroys hostile bacteria infested in the intestines. Radish-juice gives sure benefits in the burning sensation in the kidney and in urinal troubles. The juice of tender leaves of radish is useful in bile and in gynecic diseases. It vitalizes the liver and the heart. It has a beneficial effect on mucous membrane. It has a soothing effect on burning sensation.

Note : Mastication of radish leaves cures dental ailments and constipation. The mixture of carrot-juice and radish-juice makes an excellent drink. Carrot-juice makes radish-juice mild.

ALFALFA (RIJAK/RAJKO)

Introduction : Alfalfa is used as the best fodder for animals. It is considered indispensable for the health of cattle. Cows, oxen, buffaloes, horses , and other animals are nourished with alfalfa in order to make them healthy and strong. We have learnt from the west the benevolent action of alfalfa on human being.

Qualities : Alfalfa is pungent, dry and heavy. It expels gas and dislodges cough. Its juice is good for the heart.

Contents : A detailed analysis of the properties of alfalfa is not yet available. It contains valuable and useful minerals such as magnesium, phosphorus, chlorine, silicon, potassium and calcium. This alkaline grass alleviates acidity of the blood and the body.

Use : Juice can be extracted by pounding alfalfa.

Benefits : Alfalfa is good for the heart, as it energizes it. Its chlorophyll content is a powerful antiseptic. It destroys hostile germs infested in the intestines. Germs of contagious diseases are also killed by it and diseases come under control.

Note : Alfalfa-juice being very strong and pungent should normally be taken in combination with juices of other vegetables like spinach or carrots.

DRUMSTICK LEAVES (SARAGVO/SAHIJAN)

There are large trees of drumstick. Drumsticks (pods) are very popular. They are immensely used in food. But the leaves are not generally used as vegetable.

Qualities : Drumstick leaves are pungent, warm, appetizing, stimulant of gastric fire, digestive, regimen and laxative. It expels gas, intestinal worms and cough. They are very effective against eye-diseases.

Analysis of Contents

Water	75.00%
Protein	6.7%
Fat	1.7%
Carbohydrates	13.4%
Minerals	2.3%
Calcium	0.44%
Phosphorus	0.07%
Iron	7 mg/100 gm
Vitamin 'A'	11,300 I. U./100 gm
Vitamin 'B'	70 I. U./100 gm
Vitamin 'C'	220 mg/100 gm

Drumstick leaves are important because of the high vitamin 'A' content. No other leafy vegetable contains as much vitamin 'A' as drumstick leaves.

Use : Juice can ·be extracted by pounding drumstick leaves. Its juice, mixed with any other vegetable-juice, is recommended for frequent use.

Benefits : Drumstick leaves' juice mixed with honey gives benefit in internal as well as external eye-diseases. The juice mixed with sugar gives relief in colitis. Its application to hair is effective against dandruff.

DILL AS A LEAFY VEGETABLE

All of us are acquainted with dill leaves. As dill-juice expels gas, it is given to children. The medicine known as 'dill-water' is nothing but juice of dill leaves.

Qualities : As a leafy vegetable, dill is pungent, bitter, delicious and warm. It kindles gastric fire. It increases nursing mother's milk and is easy of digestion. It cures gas, colitis, windiness, cough and fever.

Contents : Like other leafy vegetables, dill also contains minerals and vitamin 'A' in considerable quantities.

Use : Dill-juice can be obtained by pounding dill leaves. Juice of dill leaves mixed with juices of other leafy vegetables is a good combination. Cooked dill leaves can be used as a vegetable item in our daily diet.

Benefits : Dill as a leafy vegetable is a sure remedy for constipation. Instead of taking fruitsalt and other laxatives one should take dill leaves (as a vegetable) with one's usual meals. It brings beneficial results. Dill leaves are very effective against piles.

***

32. THE WHEATGRASS-JUICE

"The wheatgrass-juice has been used with tremendous success for conquering cancer. It is a fail-proof remedy for rejuvenation of the body."   — Dr. Ann Wigmore

No other raw food has been acclaimed as useful as the wheatgrass. The wheatgrass-juice has not only conquered minor diseases like catarrh and cough but also fatal diseases like cancer.

Dr. Ann Wigmore, an eminent woman naturopath, can

be considered the pioneer of the wheatgrass therapy which has now become very popular. She is a staunch supporter of the wheatgrass therapy. She is of the firm opinion that the wheatgrass has an incredible curative powers. She treats all sorts of patients with wheatgrass-juice in her institute in America which is named as 'Hippocrates Health Institute'. She has written two very inspiring books 'Why Suffer' and 'Be Your Own Doctor' on this subject.

There is an interesting reference in the 'Old Testament', a holy book of the Christians : When the king lost his physical and mental health, he heard the divine voice : 'Eat the grass as an ox eats.' The king followed this divine counsel and regained his health.

Dr. Thomas, a well-known grass expert, has worked on numerous kinds of grass. He has come to a conclusion that the wheatgrass is the best of all. The wheatgrass-juice gives more and complete nourishment to the body in comparison to all other juices. It contains various kinds of abundant live minerals, vitamins and other nutrients. It contains all those substances that are in the blood of a healthy man – the difference is only of colour. The wheatgrass-juice therefore can be called green blood. Dr. Thomas has spent 50 years of his life in this research. He concluded that wheatgrass-juice has abundant medicinal properties. One can pass one's entire life by living on wheatgrass-juice. He is of the opinion that wheatgrass-juice is 'a complete food'.

Thousands of patients, whose diseases had been declared incurable by modern medicine, have been marvellously benefited by the regular use of the wheatgrass-juice and simple food.

In December 1982, at the Mumbai Hospital of Mumbai, a raw diet and wheatgrass-juice programme was carried out under the guidance of Dr. Ann Wigmore. The programme lasted for a month. Experts of modern medicine serving in the hospital admitted that the programme had bestowed unimaginable benefits to a lot of patients whose suffering could not have been allayed by medicines or surgery. It was a grand exhibition of Nature's victory over man.

Dr. Ann Wigmore has narrated in her books several miraculous and inspiring results obtained through the use of the wheatgrass-juice. It is not possible to include them all in this book. However, a few instances have been briefly given below :

①

Conquering cancer : A man of 65 years had been suffering from cancer for 14 years. He was even unable to speak. He had already tried more than a hundred remedies for the cure of this disease which included chemotherapy, radiotherapy and surgery. All these remedies had destroyed the major part of his jaw. As it was impossible for him to eat through the mouth, he was being fed by the Ryle's tube.

He had met a prominent plastic surgeon to get his deformed jaw reshaped. The surgeon expressed his helplessness saying that his cancer was of a spreading nature and had spread widely and therefore the operation would serve no purpose.

This patient, disappointed and frustrated, once came to know about the wheatgrass.

He met Dr. Wigmore on the 29th of September. At that time his deformed face looked terribly frightening and his cancer gave unbearable foul odour.

The patient was admitted to the Health Institute. The treatment started with feeding him with a glassful of the wheatgrass-juice four times a day.

At the end of the third day, that is, on 2nd October, the first symptoms of improvement became visible. The cancerous part stopped emitting foul smell.

During the second week, the regimen of the wheatgrass-juice was intensified. Besides, a piece of cloth soaked in the wheatgrass-juice was frequently kept around his throat and on the affected part of his face. Within a few days, puss ceased to flow from the two wounds on the throat.

During the third week, the patient's condition was so much improved that he began to talk a little. Thus the sun of hope peeped through the clouds of despair and frustration. Sorrow turned into joy.

During the fourth week, an improbability happened to be a fact. Old wounds on the throat began to heal gradually. After some days, they were completely healed.

On 23rd November, the patient got his body checked by modern methods. The disappearance of cancerous cells was a matter of surprise for the doctors. They could not trust their eyes. The patient bade good-bye to Dr. Wigmore with a feeling of gratitude and joy.

After some months, when he met Dr. Wigmore again, he could hardly be recognized. The deformation that had remained on his face was removed by plastic surgery. He also informed that he had been getting his old house at Pennsylvania repaired and that he had been planning for his bright future. All his plannings and programmes were the proofs of his faith that he would live long.

(2)

Leukemia (_Blood-cancer_) was also cured : In the month of August, a woman brought her husband to Dr. Wigmore. His condition was pitiable. His body was very weak and face very pale and white. He was not even able to stand.

Narrating the history of her husband's ailments, the woman said to Dr. Wigmore, _"Before a year, I had got my husband examined at Beth Israel Hospital for his debility and other ailments. At the end of various tests, it was diagnosed that my husband had been suffering from leukemia. Both of us were greatly shocked to know this. The specialists were of the_

*opinion that my husband would not be able to live more than
a year or two despite the best treatment.*

*"The shock was unbearable. My husband stopped work-
ing. In spite of medicines and careful treatment, his health
began to deteriorate. Time passed in agony. During that
period, some cancer-experts had been consulted and treatment continued. Yesterday, when I took him to the hospital,
he was so weak that he was unable even to stand, Doctors
told me in private that my husband would hardly live for a few
days. When my husband got the hint, he collapsed in the car.*

*"At night our neighbour gave me information about the
wheatgrass and almost forced me to try it. 'A drowning man
catches at a straw' and so we have come to you."*

Dr. Wigmore gave them complete information regarding
the wheatgrass and advised them to begin treatment at home.
Perhaps she might have considered the patient's condition
hopeless. Nevertheless, this treatment was started as a last
resort.

After six months, on Tuesday the 19th February, a motor-
car came and stopped in front of Dr. Wigmore's Health
Institute. A middle-aged man energetically came out of it.
Climbing the steps with agility, he rushed to Dr. Wigmore,
Extending his hand in jovial mood he asked, "Do you
recognize me, Madam?" The doctor was perplexed. Without
waiting for the doctor's reply the visitor continued, "During
the last fall my wife had brought me here. At that time I was
not even able to stand. I am the same person."

Dr. Wigmore could not at first trust his words. What a
difference! That man was white, pale and weak. This man
was full of youthful energy! His body was full of agility,
energy and vitality. His eyes were lustrous.

The visitor continued speaking, *"On that day we bade
you goodbye and returned home. My wife began to sow*

wheat at our door-step. Exactly after a weak I began to take the wheatgrass-juice. My wife gave me a cupful of wheat-grass-juice four times a day. Gradually my health began to improve. During the next six months there was a considerable improvement in my health. On 20th January we went to Beth Israel Hospital to get my body checked. The doctors who had formerly examined me were surprised and perplexed. They carefully studied and restudied my old records and stared at me in astonishment. They admitted that I was perfectly healthy but did not ask how my health improved."

After some time he heartily thanked Dr. Wigmore and took his leave.

After four months, when he met Dr. Wigmore again, his health was much more improved. There was no trace of leukemia. According to him, five cancer-experts had examined him very carefully and minutely during the last four months. They admitted that they did not understand how the miracle had happened nor were they ready to declare that wheatgrass had effected this cure. They were of the opinion that leukemia was still an incurable disease, because it was authoritatively declared so. But these experts forget that nothing is impossible for the omnipotent Nature.

From the above two instances, one should not mistakenly think that such experiments are being conducted only in foreign countries. Even in our country, many experiments on the wheatgrass have been carried out with encouraging and inspiring results.

③

A gentleman of Mumbai suffered from a strange type of illness. His body turned quite black and the skin stiff and brittle.

He was treated by eminent doctors with the medicines and injections. Various types of oils and other medicinal herbs were massaged on his body but there was no improvement.

At last under the pressure of his family and with great reluctance he consented to try the wheatgrass-juice. There was slow and gradual but definite improvement in his health. At the end of the fifteenth month, the blackness of his body disappeared completely. The hair on his hands and legs which had fallen off began to grow again. Black hair appeared on his head. Later, he began to drop the wheatgrass-juice into his eyes with the result that he was now able to read the newspaper without the help of spectacles which formerly he was unable to do. His appetite was revived and his weak body gained fresh blood. Alertness and freshness replaced fatigue and weakness. Thus in a way his body was rejuvenated.

(4)

A 22 years young woman of Anand found her hair turning prematurely white. Because of this, she started to suffer from shyness and inferiority complex. The treatment by medicines and various kinds of oils failed to help. At last, she resorted to the use of wheatgrass-juice. Within three months, her trouble vanished for ever.

(5)

A middle-aged man's case is interesting. After typhoid the condition of his body was pitiable; he had lost half of his weight, his hair began to become grey rapidly, his skin had become pale and loose and wrinkles had formed on it. He had lost his appetite and was unable to concentrate on any work on account of weakness and sluggishness. Due to these ailments, the man lost the balance of his mind. At last he gave up all kinds of treatment and turned to follow the wheatgrass-juice therapy. There was a gradual improvement in his health. Within two months, all his ailments disappeared. He gained weight by 15 lbs. His hair began to grow black. He began to feel alert and energetic. The man admitted that he had obtained a new lease of life.

* * *

In the books written by Dr. Wigmore, there are references of miraculous results obtained by the use of the wheatgrass-juice in more than 350 diseases. She states that the use of the wheatgrass can cure minor or major, old and chronic and hard-to-cure or incurable diseases. Researches are being conducted on wheatgrass simultaneously in more than 50 laboratories in America. From this, it is evident that even suspicious and conservative Europeans and Americans have found miraculous healing powers in the wheatgrass.

How to grow wheatgrass : One who has an open piece of plot to grow wheatgrass should divide it into seven parts or one can use broad-mouthed earthen pots or wooden boxes. Seven such basins are required for one individual. Fill three-fourth of the basin with black soil and one-fourth with manure. Manure should necessarily be natural (compost). Chemical fertilizers should not be used. The size of the basin should be about one square foot. 100 gm of wheat seeds should be sown in each basin. Normally 100 to 125 gm of wheatgrass grows out of this quantity.

Soak wheat-grains for twelve hours before they are sown. Then take them out of water and put them in a wet thick cloth. Bind the cloth tightly. These wheat-grains will be sprouted. If sprouted wheat-grains are sown, the height of the grass will be 5 to 7 inches within seven days.

Sprinkle water in the pot every 24 hours. Do not pour water into the pot because excess of water hinders the growth of wheat.

As there are seven earthen pots, wheat should be sown in one pot each day. The wheat sown on the first day will grow into wheatgrass and on the seventh day the wheatgrass will be of seven inches height which is necessary and ideal. This wheatgrass should be cut with scissors or pulled out manually. Wheatgrass having been taken out of the pot, soil should be removed from the pot and dried in the heat of the sun. Then a small quantity of compost manure should be added to the soil before wheatgrains are sowed again. It should be remembered that only one pot (basin) is to be prepared each day. All the seven pots are not to be simultaneously prepared.

How to extract juice : The wheatgrass having been taken out from the pot should be thoroughly washed. Then after sprinkling some water on it, it should be pounded in a domestic mortar or with a stone. Pounded wheatgrass should be put in a piece of cloth and juice can be extracted by squeezing the cloth. This method involves labour, particularly when one needs plenty of juice. Nowadays electric gadgets for extracting juice are available. Wheatgrass-juice can be extracted with ease and rapidly with the help of these gadgets.

If one does not want to extract juice, one can consume wheatgrass by chewing it. After sucking the juice, fibres should be spitted out.

Normally about 5 to 6 ounces of juice can be extracted from 100 gm. of wheatgrass. As water has been sprinkled, the juice also contains some proportion of water.

Dose and time for taking wheatgrass-juice : An average daily dose of wheatgrass-juice in moderate illness or trouble is about 100 ml (or 100 gm of wheatgrass should be masticated). The patient should begin with 25 to 50 ml of juice gradually increasing the quantity. In case of old, chronic diseases the quantity should be finally increased to 250 to 300 ml.

One should take the juice immediately after it has been extracted from wheatgrass. It should not be swallowed but should be sipped in draughts. Juice, if preserved, loses its precious ingredients. Nothing should be eaten or drunk for half an hour before or after drinking the juice.

Beginning and caution : Before one begins to take exclusive wheatgrass-juice, one should observe fast for a day or two or should live purely on fruit-juices for two or three days. Wheatgrass-juice is more effective when taken after fasting. In the initial stage one should take juice in small quantity. The quantity should be increased gradually, because some persons after taking wheatgrass-juice suffer from nausea, vomiting, cold, diarrhoea and fever. Such symptoms appear in only five to seven per cent of cases. One should not worry about such symptoms. In such cases, one should dilute the wheatgrass-juice with water. If the symptoms are persistent, one should stop taking the juice for a day or two. One should resume taking the juice when troublesome symptoms disappear. Nothing should be added to the juice for the sake of taste.

The ingredients contained in the wheatgrass-juice and their nutritive value : The wheatgrass-juice is a live food. There is a proverb : **'Life begets life'.**

As it has been stated above, Dr. Thomas considers the wheatgrass-juice to be a complete food. As per his opinion, one can live a full span of life solely on wheatgrass-juice. It means that the wheatgrass-juice contains all the ingredients required for a healthy living.

The chlorophyll contained in the wheatgrass purifies the blood and destroys hostile bacteria thriving in the intestines. The chlorophyll particles are similar to haemoglobin. So it works as an iron-element in anemia. Dr. Birscher, a research scientist, calls chlorophyll 'Concentrated sun power'. According to him, chlorophyll increases the function of the heart, beneficially affects the vascular system, the intestines, the urinary bladder and lungs. It is a unique tonic because it enhances the basic change in nitrogen.

The wheatgrass-juice contains vitamins 'A', 'B', 'E' and 'K' in a large amount. The wheatgrass contains 600 per cent more vitamin B complex than wheat.

Experts believe that wheatgrass contains an anti-cancer element called Laetrile (B_{17}) in a large amount. Dr. Laetrile Cabus says that germinated wheat-grains (wheatgrass) contain hundred times more laetrile than wheat.

Magnesium is very essential to keep the 30 enzymes in our body active. This mineral is freely available from the wheatgrass-juice.

According to Dr. Thomas's statement, 15 lbs of wheatgrass provides as much nutrition as 350 lbs of carefully chosen vegetables.

A common belief that uncooked or raw food is heavy of digestion and produces abdominal pain is absolutely groundless. It is an established fact that cooked food takes six to eight hours for complete digestion, raw food takes three to four hours, whereas vegetable and fruit-juices take only one to one and a half hours for digestion and complete absorption. Thus juices give quick nourishment.

The diseases that can be cured by the wheatgrass : The wheatgrass has been successfully used in curing the following diseases :

(1) Dermatological diseases (2) Mental and physical disorders (3) Diseases related to urinary bladder (4) Kidney-stone (5) Constipation (6) Stomach disorders (7) Diabetes (8) Heart disease (9) Disorders of joints and muscles (10) Parkinson's disease (11) Chronic cold (12) Fissure (13) Premature greying of hair (14) Gynaec diseases (15) Asthma (16) Impotence (17) Eye and ear diseases (18) Insomnia (19) Anemia (20) Cancer and certain other diseases.

Dr. Wigmore inviting the patient suffering from any disease, tells them : "Take this treatment for only twenty-one days. You will realize that new energy is overflowing in your body, nectar is being poured into your body." The wheatgrass-juice is not only a medicine but is a pot full of nectar which rejuvenates your body completely.

***

33. HONEY

"Honey is a unique medicine."

—*Ayurvedacharya Vagbhata*

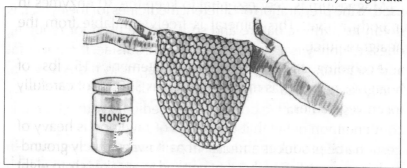

A drop of honey is, a wordless, pleasant poem, a divine song accomplishing sweet harmony, a chorus of warmth and light. Colours of innumerable flowers and their pleasant fragrance are latent in every drop of honey. Honey is a harmless combination of the perfume and sweetness of flowers.

Aristotle has stated, "When the stars rise in the sky and the rainbow is visible, pure honey oozes from the atmosphere. Honey is the sky's perspiration, or the sweet saliva dripping from the stars or the nectar trickling from the air."

There are references in the Vedas that people in those days were used to taking honey with spirituous liquor. There are eulogies on honey. In the Arabian literature, honey pervades the poetry. Honey has a unique place in the poems of Hafiz.

The value of honey has been accepted in India since time immemorial. In Egypt also, honey had been used in the preparation of various types of medicines. In ancient Greece, it was very popular. In Olympic games, it was largely used with hot water after strenuous exercises to replenish the store of exhausted energy. Hippocrates, the father of the European medicine, believed that honey bestowed long life and therefore used to recommend it to his patients.

According to Vagbhata, honey is good for eyes and is used in the preparation of different medicines for the eyes. It is dry in its intrinsic nature and so it can be used for reducing obesity. Honey is a 'rasayana'. It is aphrodisiac. It reduces fat and increases virility. It dislodges phlegm. In the Ayurveda, honey is regarded to be *'Yogavahi'* It means that honey increases the curative power of the medicine with which it is combined.

The bees suck the nectar from flowers and deposit it in their honey sack. The bees have to visit over two to five lakh flowers to gather one kg. of honey. Sometimes they fly to a distance of two miles from their hive in search of flowers. Honey stored in the hive has 75 per cent of water. But as the time passes the water evaporates to a large extent. During this process, the water content of the nectar is reduced to 20 per cent.

In reality, the nectar gathered by the bees is a form of cane-sugar, but in the honey sack of the bee it undergoes chemical changes. The cane-sugar is converted into a combination of dextrose and levulose. Hence the cane-sugar content of honey is only 1.9 per cent. The total sugar content of honey is 76.4 per cent, of which levulose forms 40.5 per cent and dextrose 34 per cent. The average percentage of other constituents is : dextrin (1.5 per cent) and ash (0.18 per cent). Besides, it contains iron, phosphorus, calcium, sodium, potassium, sulphur and manganese in small quantities. It is the darker varieties of honey which contain more mineral salts.[1] Honey contains the following vitamins in moderate quantities :

1. The U. S. A. Dept. of Agriculture–Crops in War and Peace, p. 311, Washington, 1950–51.

Thiamin 6 microgrammes, riboflavin 60 microgrammes, niacin 32 microgrammes and vitamin 'C' 5 microgrammes.

As a sweet, honey is far superior to cane-sugar. Of all the carbohydrates, it is most easily digestible.

In the Moscow hospital, on an experimental basis, T. B. patients were given 580 to 750 grams of honey daily. The patients gained weight. They obtained considerable relief from cough. Their haemoglobin percentage increased. As a fuel for the body, honey has no equal. Sugar is honey is predigested and is directly assimilable. Its absorption takes place right from the tongue.[1] As it can be assimilated without taxing the digestive organs, it constitutes an admirable food for weak persons. It has a beneficial effect on indigestion, colitis and acidity. In fever, when it is difficult to digest food, honey serves the purpose of a medicine for preserving energy. It is recommended as a good food in typhoid and pneumonia.[2]

According to Dr. J. H. Kellogg, honey is an ideal food in the heart and the liver disorders. In the case of weakness of the heart or in hysteria, if honey is given with warm water, it serves the purpose of brandy or spirit of ammonia.

Honey is full of powerful antibacterial properties. The diarrhoea germs when placed in honey could not survive for more than 10 hours. The paratyphoid and the typhoid germs died within 24 and 48 hours respectively.[3]

Ulcers heal rapidly when honey is applied to them. Honey is a mild laxative. It cures constipation and gives relief in cold, cough and sore throat. It is helpful in disturbed urination. It is considered to be a remedy for rheumatism and arthritis.

* * *

1. A. I. Root–The ABC and XYZ of Bee Culture, The A. I. Root Company, Media, 1950
2. Bodog F. Beck, M.D. and Doree Smedly, Honey and Your Health, pp. 120–155, New York
3. A. I. Root–The ABC and XYZ of Bee Culture

34. REJUVENATION BY MILK

Milk is a complete food. Milk contains all the nutrients necessary for the body. Milk is the nectar on the earth.

Expert dietitians agree that the milk fresh from the cow makes an excellent diet provided the cow is healthy and is given proper fodder and proper cleanliness is maintained at the time of milking it. Fresh milk means warm milk from the udder. Vagbhat has also compared the milk fresh from the cow with nectar and has ascribed many virtues to it.

Milk increases strength. It is easy of digestion. It has a cooling effect. It is stimulant and a curative agent in all the three principal ailments (windiness, bile and cough).

Only milk fresh from the udder of the cow can be taken directly. If it is kept even for a short while, one should take it only after warming it. Where proper cleanliness is doubted, one should take it only after boiling it.

Under the circumstances stated above, milk is considered to be the best diet. It contains all the nutrients necessary for the human body. One can get the maximum benefit of this complete diet only when it is regularly taken. Milk taken with other food loses many of its benefits. This is why milk-cure has a special significance.

The distinction between milk-diet and milk-cure (rejuvenation by milk) should be clearly understood. In milk-diet one can take as much milk as one can without abandoning one's regular food, while in milk-cure only milk is taken regularly in a planned way.

The eminent Dr. Kellogg[1] of America writes, "Milk-diet can be useful to those whose aim is to increase their weight.

---

1. Dr. Kellogg J. H., M. D.–The New Dietetics, Modern Medicine Publishing Co., Washington

But excessive milk-diet with other food is injurious to the digestive process. On the other hand, planned milk-cure is beneficial in many diseases. Milk-cure eliminates digestive disorders.

The large intestine contains bacteria which cause putrefaction or fermentation. When milk is consumed with other food, these bacteria putrefy milk and cause fermentation in it. This leads to disorders relating to the digestion. But those who subsist purely on milk suffer no such disorders. The reasons are as follows :

(1) If milk is taken in large quantity, its calcium content and other mineral salts contained in it check the acidity in the stomach. Besides, the efficacy of reagin, an enzyme oozing in the stomach is reduced with the result that small quantities of split milk in stomach become smooth.

(2) If an exclusive milk-diet is taken in a large quantity, its lactose directly reaches the intestines and inactivates the bacteria which cause fermentation and putrefaction in the intestines. When a patient is kept on an exclusive milk-diet, he is made to take about 6 litres of milk during the latter half of the treatment period out of which 500 grams of lactose directly reaches the intestines. Dr. Rissiyar and Dr. Martley have proved that even if one per cent of lactose reaches the large intestine, activities of hostile bacteria can be checked.

The chemical analysis of milk shows that milk contains the following nutrients :

Water	87.2%
Fat	3.9%
Lactose	3.75%
Protein	3.40%
Minerals	0.75%

The mineral salts contained in milk include calcium phosphate, potassium phosphate, sodium chloride, potassium chloride, iron phosphate, manganese phosphate, etc. Milk also contains a lot of vitamins 'A', 'B', 'D' and 'E' and some vitamin 'C'.

Milk-cure or Rejuvenation by milk : Milk has been used as a curative agent since ancient times. The patients disappointed with other remedial methods have been benefited by milk-cure. During the last few years, milk-cure has been widely recognized in America also.

The protein of milk is of highest biological value and easy of digestion. It contains all the amino-acids necessary for the body. The iron-content of milk is not large. However, since a large amount of milk is consumed during milk-cure, the body's requirements of iron are satisfied. The milk contains all the ingredients necessary for the body.

Pre-requisites for milk-cure : It is essential to make certain preparations before starting milk-cure or milk-treatment. Without them one does not get expected benefits. First of all the patient should try simple and harmless natural remedies (nature-cure) for the cure of his disease. Milk-cure should begin after the disease comes under control.

Before the patient begins milk-cure, he should keep on an alkaline diet (fruits, vegetables, juices) for a few days. This strengthens the base (foundation) of health. A solid building of good health can be constructed on such a rock foundation through milk-cure.

Method of milk-cure : Prior to milk-diet therapy, one should observe fast for four days, and then should take milk, after every two hours for first six days as per the chart given below :

Day	Dose	How many times?	Total quantity of milk to be taken
First	25 ml	7 times	175 ml
Second	50 ml	7 times	350 ml
Third	75 ml	7 times	525 ml
Fourth	100 ml	7 times	700 ml
Fifth	125 ml	7 times	875 ml
Sixth	150 ml	7 times	1050 ml

(**Note** : From the seventh day milk should be taken at the intervals of
one and a half hours instead of two hours.)

Day	Dose	How many times?	Total quantity of milk to be taken
Seventh	150 ml	9 times	1350 ml
Eighth	170 ml	9 times	1575 ml
Ninth and Tenth	200 ml	9 times	1800 ml

(**Note** : From the eleventh day milk should be taken at the intervals of
one hour instead of one and a half hours.)

Day	Dose	How many times?	Total quantity
Eleventh	200 ml	12 times	2400 ml
Twelfth	250 ml	12 times	3000 ml
Thirteenth	300 ml	12 times	3600 ml

From the fourteenth day 300 ml of milk should be taken
at the intervals of 45 minutes, for sixteen times a day. Do not
take milk one time at noon. Thus the total quantity of milk to
be taken during the day will be about 5 litres. This order, dose
and quantity should be continued for at least forty days.

The first dose of milk should be taken at seven in the
morning and the last dose should be taken at seven in the
evening. As milk already contains sufficient quantity of sugar,
no extra sugar should be added to it.

The above-mentioned table is prepared after cautious
scrutiny. Start slowly. It is desirable that milk should be taken
in small quantity in the beginning. Nevertheless if one's
digestive power is very good, one can take approximately 100
ml of milk each time. Thus one can consume 7 to 8 litres of
milk each day.

Five litres of milk consumed strictly according to the
guideline produces 3600 calories. Out of these 3600 calories,
1700 calories are obtained from fat, 800 from protein and
1100 from lactose.

The method of taking milk : Expert dieticians advise us to chew milk instead of drinking it. By sipping the milk slowly in draughts saliva secreted in the mouth mixes with it, with the result that digestion of lactose starts right from the mouth. Milk swallowed does not digest properly.

The quality of milk and the process to be made on it : Usually, for rejuvenation, cow milk is consumed.[1] Fresh cow milk is not available in cities. So it is advisable to boil milk. A single overbrim is enough. Then, whenever milk is to be taken, it should be warmed a little. For this, a glass of milk should be put in hot water for a few minutes.

Important instructions : During the milk-diet, treatment some physical disorders or disturbances may arise. The milk-diet experimentation requires proper understanding and pre-planning on the part of one who wishes to adopt the treatment. Sometimes abdominal troubles creep up. Constipation, if any, should be cured by enema. If one suffers from diarrhoea because of milk, the dose should be reduced for a day or two. Another way is that fat should be removed from milk before it is consumed (skimmed milk) or milk should be diluted by adding some water. There is another good alternative that is to take a date or two with milk.

If one suffers from nausea sensation or vomiting, one should take lemon-juice. After each dose of milk (or whenever necessary), sucking a piece of lemon gives a relief. Lemon-juice can also be mixed with orange or mozambique-juice. Sucking ice-pieces quietens vomit-sensation and vomiting. During milk-cure therapy, some patients suffer from swollen gums, bodyache or fever. One need not worry for these symptoms. In the case of swollen gums, one should gargle with warm water mixed with salt. In case of fever, one should stop taking milk and observe fast for a day or two. When the temperature of the body comes down, resume milk again.

---

1. If available goat-milk can also be taken.

Sometimes is happens that, during milk-diet treatment, certain old, suppressed diseases surface suddenly. It should be remembered that, during milk-diet treatment, the body makes strenuous efforts to eliminate toxic foreign elements from it. The consequence is that the toxic elements lying dormant in the body try to come out of the tissues and hence the symptoms of diseases appear. This is a critical time (not dangerous or harmful). If the patient is not aware of the fact, he is frightened. But experts take these symptoms as inevitable and necessary. According to them, when these symptoms subside of their own, it is a sign that the body is completely cleansed. The health regained, after the body is completely cleansed, is pure and stable.

Many naturopaths recommend hot-water bath or tub-bath during milk-diet treatment. Such a bath stimulates the glands of perspiration and eliminates toxic elements rapidly. Moreover, the blood circulation gets impetus. In milk-diet therapy, a hot-water bath is very beneficial.

During milk-diet treatment, the patient should try to conserve his energy. He must take complete rest.

The completion of milk-diet therapy : Milk-diet treatment should be brought to an end after 40 or more days. On the final day, milk should be consumed only till noon. In the afternoon, fruits, fruit-juice or vegetable-juice should be taken. The next day, also milk should be taken only for half a day. In the afternoon fruits, whereas, in the evening boiled vegetables should be taken. On the third day, milk should be taken in the morning, at noon and in the evening. In between, fruits and boiled vegetables should be taken. From the fourth day, a small quantity of cooked food should be taken and then the quantity should be increased gradually to reach the usual simple diet.

Benefits of milk-cure : Milk-diet has no equal for one who desires to increase one's weight. There is visible increase in weight as early as two or three days after the commencement of milk-diet treatment. The gain in weight is not due to an increase in fat, but due to the formation of new, firm muscle-tissue. The ailments like shrunken eyes, wrinkled skin and deformed abdomen are eliminated by milk-cure therapy. As milk-cure progresses, the eyes become clean and shining and the face becomes radiant.

Dr. Bernarr McFadden writes that milk-cure has a benevolent effect on the blood-circulation. Slow-going and weak pulses become vitalized and quick.[1]

The rapid circulation of blood eliminates numbness from the arms and the legs and produces warmth in them.

Exclusive milk-diet gives benefits in kidney-diseases. The lactose and other elements contained in milk are easy of digestion. Hence the digestive system gets relief. The lactose contained in milk destroys undesirable (hostile) bacteria which produce putrefaction and fermentation of food in the intestines. On the other hand, it (lactose) increases the number of bacteria which are useful to the body.

Milk-diet therapy cleanses the body completely making it free from harmful elements. So it is beneficial to nearly all the diseases.

It is very essential that the patients suffering from obesity, cold, high blood pressure, cardiac trouble and diabetes should undertake milk-cure therapy under the guidance of an expert naturopath. One should take extreme care before adopting milk-diet treatment when one is suffering from the chronic diseases of the liver and the gall bladder. To such patients thick buttermilk-diet (lassi) is very congenial and favourable. Thick-buttermilk-diet therapy is discussed in the next chapter.

* * *

---

1. Dr. Bernarr McFadden : Home Health Library, p. 1373

35. REJUVENATION BY THICK BUTTERMILK

Many expert dietieians consider thick buttermilk(matha) to be more effective than milk or curd in certain ailments. Thick buttermilk has a special significance as it is light and easy of digestion. It is called the nectar of the earth. It has no equal in rejuvenating the body by expelling harmful elements from it.

The properties and effects of buttermilk vary in proportion to the quality of milk of which it is made. If one desires to get oneself rejuvenated by thick buttermilk, one should use only the milk of cow. A mixture of three-fourths of curd with one-fourth of water makes a delicious thick buttermilk. The sour curd should not be used for preparing buttermilk. For treatment, thick buttermilk should be prepared three to four times from fresh curd three to four times every day.

There is a clear reference in 'Bhavaprakash', the famous ancient book of medicine, that one who takes thick buttermilk in the prescribed manner never loses one's health.

According to the Ayurveda, thick (cow) buttermilk is delicious, light and warm. It kindles gastric fire. It is sweet and digestive. It eliminates all the three principal systemic disturbances i.e., 'vata', 'pitta' and 'cough'. It helps to digest fried items, sweets, and other heavy items.

Thick buttermilk made of skim-milk is nearly devoid of fat. Other contents of thick buttermilk are as follows :

Protein	about 3.2 to 3.4	per cent
Lactose	about 4.6 to 5.2	per cent
Lactic acid	about 0.5 to 1.1	per cent
Calcium	about 0.12 to 0.14	per cent
Phosphorus	about 0.09 to 0.1	per cent
Iron	about 0.2 to 0.3	per cent

It also contains magnesium, potassium, sodium, chlorine, sulphur and other salts in small proportion. It contains vitamin 'B$_2$' 30 mg/100 gm and vitamin 'A' in a small quantity.

The method of taking thick buttermilk for rejuvenation : The method of taking thick buttermilk for rejuvenation is the same as that of taking milk. If taking milk for rejuvenation does not suit one, one can take thick buttermilk instead. It should be well remembered that thick buttermilk should not be sour.

One who takes up thick buttermilk for rejuvenation in order to maintain health and to allay minor disorders need not do any pre-planning. One can begin the regimen of thick buttermilk. First of all, the patient should resort to three days.

However, in cases of chronic diseases, the patient can pre-plan to get the maximum benefit out of the regimen of thick buttermilk. First of all, the patient should resort to nature-cure to check the disease. Then he should get his body cleansed by observing fast or juice-fast for about four days. He should begin taking thick buttermilk on the fifth day. As per the chart given below, thick buttermilk should be taken every two hours.

Day	Quantity of thick buttermilk to be taken	How many times?	Total quantity of thick buttermilk
First	25 ml	7 times	175 ml
Second	50 ml	7 times	350 ml
Third	75 ml	7 times	525 ml
Fourth	100 ml	7 times	700 ml
Fifth	125 ml	7 times	875 ml
Sixth	150 ml	7 times	1050 ml

Note : From the 7th day onwards, thick buttermilk should be taken at the intervals of 1½ hours instead of 2 hours.

Day	Quantity of thick buttermilk to be taken	How many times?	Total quantity of thick buttermilk
Seventh	150 ml	9 times	1350 ml
Eighth	175 ml	9 times	1575 ml
Ninth and Tenth	200 ml	9 times	1800 ml

Note : From the eleventh day, thick buttermilk should be taken at the interval of one hour.

Eleventh	200 ml	12 times	2400 ml
Twelfth	250 ml	12 times	3000 ml
Thirteenth	300 ml	12 times	3600 ml

From the fourteenth day, the patient should take thick buttermilk at the intervals of every three quarters of an hour and sixteen times a day. Thick buttermilk should not be taken in noon time. This order should be continued at least for 30 days. Some experts advise to continue the regimen for even more days.

Start should be made by taking the first dose in the morning at 7. Buttermilk should be taken till 7 in the evening. Neither sugar nor salt should be added to it for taste. Adjustments in quantity, if circumstances warrant, may be undertaken.

The conclusion of the regimen of thick buttermilk : The patient should take thick buttermilk six times (only for the first half of the day) on the day when the regimen is to be concluded. In the afternoon, he should take fruits of vegetables or whole fruits containing minimum quantity of fibres. The same quantity of thick buttermilk should be taken on the second day but at noon he should take fruits and steamed vegetables. On the third day, he should take thick buttermilk in the morning, at noon and in the evening – three times only.

He should take fruits or steamed vegetables during the intervals. From the fourth day, he should begin taking a small quantity of cooked food. Gradually he should come back to normal diet.

Hints : During the regimen of thick buttermilk, it is possible that one may suffer from minor ailments like swelling of gums, bodyache, constipation or diarrhoea. The patient need not worry about these disorders. Sometimes, the patient feels feverish during the regimen of thick buttermilk. In such cases, he should stop taking thick buttermilk for a day or two and observe fasting. When temperature becomes normal, he should resume taking the regimen. During the regimen, there is an increase in the amount of perspiration and urine. It is natural. The patient need not worry about it.

Diseases in which thick buttermilk regimen is useful : Physicians are of the opinion that there is no remedy superior to thick buttermilk for the cure of abdominal disorders and dysentery. Thick buttermilk vitalizes, strengthens and activates the digestive organs.

Moreover, the efficacy of the regimen of thick buttermilk in skin-diseases, piles, dropsy, asthma, arthritis, diabetes and other diseases has been well established.

In short, thick buttermilk is a simple and harmless remedy for cleansing the body, expelling hostile elements from the body and for the rejuvenation of the body.

* * *

PART 3

1. JUICE-TREATMENT IN DIFFERENT DISEASES

One who wishes to resort to juice-treatment is advised to contact an expert in this subject. It is desirable that juice-treatment should be carried on under the guidance and advice of an expert.

The usefulness of juice-treatment for some common diseases has been described in this chapter. Juices cleanse the blood, expel toxic and other harmful elements from the body, prevent degeneration of the body and procure ingredients necessary for the reformation and regeneration of the cells of the body. That is why either independently or in conjunction with other modes of treatment juices give sure benefit in almost all diseases.

There are several definite reasons for the cause of diseases over and above improper food-habits. A disease cannot completely be cured unless such reasons are warded off or prevented. For example, if one is under the treatment for cold but continues to take cold eatables, or does not protect oneself from violent cold winds and rain, it is not possible to get oneself cured of cold.

Juice-treatment does not claim to be the only remedy for every disease. It is a fact which can be well understood that in the cases of some diseases and specially when it is serious one, one has to take the help of other therapies. If a certain therapy has been proven useful and effective in a particular disease, there is no reason why one should be deprived of the benefit of that therapy. For instance, hip-bath gives benefit in most of the abdominal diseases. One must not hesitate to accept this sort of treatment. The purpose of every therapy or physician is the same – to cure the disease completely and as soon as possible.

It is necessary to comprehend the disease thoroughly before the commencement of the treatment. Juice-treatment should then be planned and finally the plan should be implemented with regularity, perseverance and zeal.

Acidity : Take a mixture of juices of cabbage and carrot. In addition to it, one can take juices of cucumber, potato, apple, mosambi and watermelon. Milk also should be taken. Avoid chillies, fried food and sweets.

Acne : Take a mixture of carrot and spinach-juices. Take a mixture of juices of potato, beet-root, cucumber and grapes. Watermelon and papaya-juice may also be taken. Massage papaya or potato-juice on the face. Vapour-bath is advantageous. Do not allow greasiness to remain on the face. Aviod using cosmetics.

Anaemia : Mixed juices of leafy vegetables, juice of alfalfa and juices of beet-root, cabbage, bitter-gourd, apricot and grapes are useful in this disease.

Aphthae : First of all abdominal disorders, if any, should be cured. Constipation should be relieved. Juices of pot-herb (spinach) and cabbage should be taken.

Asthma : Take mixed juices of carrot, beet-root and cabbage. Take a mixture of juices of leafy vegetables or a mixture of juices of potato and apple. Besides, garlic and papaya juices can also be taken.

Bronchitis : Take warm water with ginger, honey and lemon-juice in the morning or, take warm water with garlic and onion-juices. Besides, take juices of radish, cabbage, beet-root, cucumber and carrot. Avoid smoking.

Cancer : Opinions are divided as to which juice gives the maximum benefit in cancer. Normally these juices are beneficial : Juices of carrot, grape, beet-root, apple, ginger, papaya, tomato and wheatgrass. One should try to maintain the health of the liver. Magnet therapy might prove useful.

Cardiac troubles : Take honey, coconut water and juices of papaya, pomegranate, pineapple and garlic.

Cholera : Juice of beelee fruit mixed with juices of mint, garlic and onion should be taken with warm water. Coconut water is very much useful in cholera.

Cold : Lemonated warm water should be taken. Juices of ginger, orange, carrot, radish, garlic, etc. can also be taken. Water-vapour is also useful.

Colitis : Take a mixture of carrot and spinach-juices. Juices of cucumber, apple, beet-root, papaya, beelee and orange are also beneficial.

Constipation : In this disease, raw whole fruits and vegetables are as beneficial as their juices. Proper exercises should be done. One should form regular habits of evacuating bowels. One should take a mixture of juices of spinach and carrot or a mixture of juices of potato, cucumber and apple. One can also take juices of fig, beelee (eagle marmaloss), guava and orange.

Contagious diseases : Take on an empty stomach a glassful of lukewarm water mixed with lemon-juice and a teaspoonful of honey. Take a glassful water mixed with a teaspoonful each of garlic and onion-juices. A mixture of carrot and mosambi-orange juices can also be taken.

Cough : Take warm water mixed with honey and lemon-juice in the morning. Also take a glassful of carrot-juice added with a tablespoonful each of garlic, onion and basil-juices.

Avoid smoking. If the disease is grave, special treatment is necessary.

Diabetes : Juices of rose-apple, tomato, cucumber,

lemon, bitter-gourd, carrot, spinach, cabbage and French bean should be taken.

Diarrhoea : Take juices of beelee fruit, apple, garlic and green turmeric. Juices of beet-root and pineapple are also recommended. Take complete rest.

Diphtheria : It requires immediate medical treatment. Take pineapple-juice and turn it over and over in the mouth before swallowing it. Take warm water mixed with garlic and onion-juices.

Dysentery : Regimen of thick buttermilk is one of the best antidotes to dysentery. Pomegranate-juice is also effective. Rose-apple juice gives benefit in this disease.

Eczema : Take a mixture of juices of carrot and spinach with juice of mixed leafy vegetables. Juices of potato, papaya and watermelon can also be taken. Besides that, potato-juice may be rubbed externally on the affected skin.

Eyes : Though vitamin 'A' is very important for the eyes, other vitamins are also equally important. One should take juices which contain all the vitamins and calcium. A mixture of carrot-juice and juices of various leafy vegetables is beneficial to the eyes. Reduce the intake of sugar.

Fever : As solid food should not be taken in fever, there is no other alternative to juices for maintaining energy. Take warm water mixed with honey and lemon-juice in the morning. Warm water with garlic and onion-juices can also be taken. Besides, take juices of cabbage, gourd, basil, pomegranate, orange and mosambi. Complete rest is essential.

For beautifying complexion : These juices are recommended for beautifying complexion : Tomato and turmeric-juices, mixed juices of beet-root and apple, guava and papaya-juices. Cucumber-juice should be drunk as well as applied externally to the skin.

For freshness and cooling : Take juices of watermelon, pineapple and apple.

Fracture : First of all, one should get his fracture treated by an orthopaedic surgeon. Afterwards, for the rapid calcification of the bone, one should follow the treatment given below :

A blend of six juices : alfalfa, spinach, pot-herb, fenugreek, drumstick and bishop's seed should be taken.

Juices of amla, watermelon, carrot, guava and papaya should also be taken. The affected part should be given proper rest. Food containing sufficient protein should be taken.

Gastric ulcers : Take about 450 ml of cabbage-juice daily. Besides, take juices of cucumber, papaya and potato. Milk can also be taken. Avoid taking citrus fruits. This ailment is mostly due to mental stress and tension. If it is so, get rid of the cause of such stress or tension. Take absolutely simple food with the minimum condiments. Avoid taking fibrous eatables.

Gout : Take warm water mixed with honey and lemon-juice. A tablespoonful of each of garlic and onion-juices can also be taken with warm water. The patient suffering from gout should particularly take the juices of French beans and cherry. Potato-juice is also useful. Avoid taking wine, non-vegetarian diet and food with excessive protein.

Headache : Take ginger-juice. Juices of carrot, beet-root, cucumber, tomato, cabbage and apple can also be taken.

High blood-pressure : Juices of garlic, basil and wheat-grass are beneficial. Juices of carrot, beet-root, cucumber, papaya, alfalfa and orange can also be taken. Avoid taking fat-saturated items like butter, ghee, vegetable-ghee, etc.

Hypercholesterolaemia (Abnormally high level of cho-lesterol in the blood) : Basil-juice as well as garlic and onion-juices are effective. Avoid taking substances which contain saturated fatty acids.

Impurity of blood : Take mixed juices of carrot and

spinach. Juices of cabbage, beet-root, tomato, lemon, apple and bitter-gourd can also be taken. A tablespoonful of green turmeric juice is proved to be useful.

Indigestion : Juice of a lemon in a glass of warm water should be taken on an empty stomach in the morning. Take a spoonful of ginger-juice half an hour before meals. Juices of papaya, pineapple, cucumber and cabbage should also be taken. A blend of juices of carrot, beet-root and spinach should be taken. Avoid overeating and do some physical exercise.

Infertility : It is necessary to find out the cause of infertility. Juices of amla, carrot, spinach, apple, tomato and such other fruits and vegetables containing vitamin 'E' should be taken. Wheatgrass-juice should also be taken.

Influenza : Take warm water mixed with honey and lemon-juice in the morning, or, take warm water mixed with garlic and onion-juices. Juices of carrot, orange and mosambi can also be taken.

Insomnia : A mixture of apple, peru (guava) and potato-juices and a mixture of carrot and spinach-juices should be taken. Juice should not be taken after 6 p.m.

Internal Haemorrhage : Take juices of apple, lemon and carrot.

Jaundice : A glassful of bitter-gourd (karela) should be taken on an empty stomach in the morning. Moreover, a mixture of juices of gourd, carrot, beet-root, cucumber and apple should be taken. A mixture of juices of papaya, green turmeric, grapes, orange and mosambi can also be taken. Chewing sugarcane pieces is very effective. Take fat-free food and avoid taking alcoholic drinks.

Kidney stone/s : Take juices of carrot, cucumber, beet-root, apple and pumpkin. Coconut water is also beneficial. Avoid taking juice of leafy vegetables. Magnetized water is very effective against kidney stones.

Loss of appetite : Lemonated water should be taken in the morning. In addition to this juices of bitter-gourd, carrot and ginger can also be taken. Constipation should be relieved. Physical exercise should be done.

Menstrual disorders : Take the juices of carrot, papaya, pineapple and grapes. Mixed juices of leafy vegetables can also be taken.

Migraine : Take a glassful water mixed with lemon-juice and a spoonful of ginger-juice.

Perform Shakasana for 15 minutes twice a day without fail.

Nausea and Vomiting : There are a number of causes of this ailment (sickness). If it is due to improper or excess eating and drinking, observe fast for a day. Take juices of pomegranate, papaya, lemon, orange, pineapple and tomato.

Nervous disorders : Juices of green leafy vegetables and french beans are useful.

Obesity : See 'Weight'.

Osteoporosis : Take food rich in calcium, vitamins 'D' and 'C' and protein. Take freely leafy vegetables, raddish, cabbage and sprouted pulses.

Peptic ulcers : Excessive secretion of hydrochloric acid in the stomach adversely affects mucous membranes and causes peptic ulcers. The cause of excessive secretion of hydrochloric acid is mostly mental tension or worries.

Cabbage-juice is a capital remedy for duodenal and peptic ulcers. One should take 400-450 ml of cabbage-juice everyday. Juices of cucumber, papaya and potato can also be taken in addition to cabbage-juice. Juice of citrous (citrus) fruits should not be taken.

Piles : Take juices of carrot, potato, fig and leafy vege- tables. Onion-juice is an excellent remedy for oozing piles.

Take fibrous food in proper quantity.

Pneumonia : Take immediate medical treatment. Take warm water with ginger, lemon and honey or take warm water with garlic and onion-juices. Juices of basil, mosambi, orange and carrot are also recommended.

Pregnancy : Take particular care to have enough of vitamins 'A', 'D' and 'C' and of iron. Take freely juices of carrot, tomato, apple, fig, beet-root, gourd and leafy vegetables.

Problems regarding teeth : Take juices of carrot, apple, guava, orange and leafy vegetables. Chew leafy vegetables. Lemon-juice is also useful. Minimize the use of sugar.

Prostate gland troubles : Pumpkin juice is an excellent remedy for these troubles. Beet-root-juice is also recommended along with pumpkin-juice.

Pyorrhoea : Masticate properly carrot, guava and apple before eating and also take their juices. Juices of lemon, orange and leafy vegetables have also proved useful. Occasionally make use of garlic and onion-juices.

Rejuvenation : All juices are useful for rejuvenation of the body. Yet, one should take plenty of juices of carrot, orange and spinach. A regimen of wheatgrass-juice should be resorted to once a year. The Ayurveda has given much importance to 'amla' which can also be very useful.

Renal diseases : All fruits are diuretic. So they give relief in the burning sensation in the kidney and in urinal disorders. However, juices particularly of beet-root, carrot, cucumber, melon, watermelon, grapes and pineapple should be taken. Furthermore, coconut water should be freely taken.

Rheumatism : Take juices of carrot, cucumber, cabbage, grapes, bitter-gourd, apple and coconut. Wheatgrass is also useful.

Scurvy : This disease is caused because of the deficiency of vitamin 'C'. Juices of citrus and sweet fruits like amla, guava, alfalfa, radish, papaya, potato, lemon, oranges, mosambi, pineapple, cherry, etc. should be taken.

Skin-diseases : Take mixed juices of carrot and spinach. Juices of potato, beet-root, cucumber, turmeric, watermelon, guava, apple, mosambi and papaya are also recommended. Potato and papaya-juice can be externally applied to the affected part of the skin.

Splenomegaly : Papaya juice is most effective in this disease. In addition to it, juices of rose-apple, lemon, green turmeric, garlic, onion and carrot should be taken.

Sun-stroke : Juices of amla and tamarind, juices of orange and mosambi, mixed or separate juices of melon and watermelon should be taken.

Throat troubles : Take warm water with honey and lemon-juice in the morning. Take a draught of pineapple-juice and turn it over and over in the mouth before swallowing it. Besides, take a mixture of juices of carrot, beet-root and cucumber. Take a glassful of warm water mixed with a spoonful each of ginger, garlic and onion-juices. A tablespoon green turmeric-juice is also useful.

Tuberculosis : Necessary medical treatment should be taken. Do not neglect the treatment. Carrot-juice is very useful. In addition to it, take juices of garlic, onion and honey.

Typhoid : Take a glassful of warm water mixed with honey and lemon-juice in the morning or take a glassful of warm water mixed with a tablespoonful each of garlic and onion-juices. Besides, a mixture of juices of pomegranate, mosambi, orange and basil-juice is also recommended.

Weakened sexual drive : Juices of these fruits and vegetables are recommended. Carrot and spinach (mixed); beetroot, cucumber and apple (mixed); pumpkin, etc. (For further information see page Nos. 28 to 30.)

Weight : To reduce the weight, take juices of carrot, cucumber and tomato.

Decrease the quantity of food. Physical exercise should be done. To increase the weight, rejuvenation by milk is most effective. In addition to it, take dry fruits. Take fruit-juices.

Worms (in gastric tract) : Add a tablespoonful of garlic-juice to a glassful of warm water. To it mix a tablespoonful of onion-juice. This mixture is very useful to one who suffers from worms. Pumpkin-juice is also beneficial. Besides these juices, a mixture of juices of fenugreek and mint and papaya-juice can also be taken.

———————

2. BLENDS OF JUICES FOR PLEASURE

The purpose of this book is to show therapeutic use of juices. Yet, it is not out of place to consider the delights of juices and their blends which energise the body and satisfy the palate. Some juices such as juices of pineapple, mosambi, orange, carrot, apple, papaya, etc. are delicious on their own. But once you have a juicer, do spend some time experimenting with blends to suit your relish and contentment.

Some excellent blends of juices are given below. In addition to them, you can make other combinations to suit your taste.

(1) **Orange-Mosambi** : Add a cupful mosambi-juice to a cupful orange-juice. Add some ice to it and enjoy the drink.

(2) **Ginger-Apple-Cherry** : Make a mixture of a cupful apple-juice, half a cupful cherry-juice and two spoonfuls ginger-juice. Add some ice to it and enjoy the drink.

(3) **Apricot-Apple** : Soak a few dried apricots in water. When they are completely soaked, remove their seeds. Put seedless apricots in a juicer. Add a few slices of an apple to it and extract juice. Add ice to it. Enjoy the taste of the combination.

(4) **Plum-Apple** : Take equal quantities of plums and apples and extract their juice with the help of a juicer. This blend delights the mind.

(5) **Pineapple-Grapes** : Extract juice from a cupful-grapes and a medium size of a pineapple slice. Add a spoonful honey and some ice to it. This combination is worth enjoying.

(6) **Carrot-Tomato-Spinach** : Extract juice from a mixture of three to four carrots, spinach and two tomatoes.

Add juice of half a lemon to it. Add some rock salt to it and the combination will be very delicious. (Do not use rock-salt in case of illness.)

(7) With the help of a juicer, extract juice from a cupful grapes (black), some pineapple and a fig. Add some ice to it. This combination is unique in taste.

(8) **Cock-tail :** Take pineapple, mosambi and apples of equal proportion and extract juice from them. Add minutely thrashed ice to it. Enjoy the drink and get refreshed.

---

3. SOME CASES SHOWING SUCCESSFUL EXPERIMENTATION OF JUICE-DIET

At times, juice-treatment is applied as an auxiliary treatment along with other treatments. When the patient begins to get relief from illness, it is difficult to know what individual contribution juice-treatment and other treatments gave to the relief. However, there are innumerable cases which were cured solely by juice-treatment. There are instances in which juice-treatment was successful, while other treatments had failed. Below are presented such interesting instances without exaggeration.

①

Two years back, a middle-aged man came to consult me for his ailment. From his appearance he looked healthy.

He stated that his ailment started with the difficulty while passing urine. Later, the trouble went on increasing. Furthermore, he was suffering from excessive sexual drive. Before he came to me, he had consulted various specialists and got himself treated by them. Doctors had diagnosed that his prostate gland was enlarging. They advised him to get the gland removed by surgery. But he was not prepared for surgery.

I advised him to apply magneto therapy and perform certain yogic asanas along with juice-diet. I prescribed him the following programme :

(1) **At 7 in the morning :** To take a glassful mixed juices of pumpkin and cucumber.

(2) **At 11 in the morning :** To take half a glassful beet-root juice.

(3) **Between 3-4 in the afternoon :** To take a glassful mixed juices of carrot and beet-root.

(4) At 7 in the evening : To take a glassful mixed juices of pumpkin and cucumber.

I suggested him to come to me on alternate days for magnetic treatment. But the man did not turn up for a long time. He again came to me after one and a half months. He delightfully told me that he got himself completely relieved from troubles. He expressed his sorrow for his inability to come to me for magnetic treatment. He stated that he had firmly and faithfully followed juice-treatment as per my instructions.

After a few months, the man came again to see me. He stated that he was still following.juice-treatment to some extent. He informed me that the surgeon who had previously examined him and advised him for an operation was very much astonished when he examined him again, and stated that no operation was necessary. The surgeon told him that his prostate gland had regained its normal size.

In the above instance, the patient was relieved of his ailment solely by juice-treatment.

(2)

A thrilling article 'A Man's Fight Against Cancer' written by Mr. Robert Stickle was published in March, 1976 issue of a periodical named 'Natural Food And Farming'. The details of the article are briefly narrated below :

Before six years, Mr. Stickle was diagnosed as suffering from 'malignant melanoma' (a kind of cancer). The cancer had developed on a large scale and had spread to many parts of the body multiple metastases. Mr. Stickle was given every kind of prevalent treatment. Chemotherapy and radio-therapy had heavily worn away his body. His health was gradually deteriorating. The doctors feared that he would probably not see the coming of the year 1971. At last, this disappionted and frustrated gentleman turned to naturopathy. He began taking juice-diet. He gradually increased the quantity of intake of juices and finally started consuming five litres of various juices during the day. Juices included those of carrot, beet-root, grapes, wheatgrass and alfalfa. There was slow but definite improvement in Mr. Stickle's health. On gaining weight and energy, he became active again. He has been leading a fully active life till today. This is indeed a miracle of juice-treatment.

3

A few days ago, I had a chance to meet a young industrialist. This industrialist had been suffering from mental stress and tension on account of intense business competition, shortage of funds, labour problems, etc. Furthermore, he had been suffering from gastric ulcers caused by his improper and irregular eating and drinking habits.

Antacids and a change in food-items gave him some relief. But this relief was purely temporary frequently suffered from pain and burning sensation in the stomach so severe that he was unable even to sleep at night. Blood was found in his stool. In short, he was perturbed and very weak.

He requested me to suggest a remedy, if any, for his ailment.

I advised him to take simple food and in addition it recommended him to take raw cabbage juice in a small quantity five times a day. In that way, he had to take a half to three quarters of a litre cabbage-juice during the day. I also suggested that he should take papaya-juice and raw potato-juice in between the intervals. I gave him instructions regarding remedies for mental tension also.

After a week, he telephoned me to inform that he was feeling much better. Though this young man who was very fond of delicious food disliked the taste of cabbage and potato-juices, he began taking these juices with zeal when he found that his health was improving. Later, he even started liking the taste of those juices.

After a few days, he personally came to see me. All his ailments were nearly over. He was so much impressed by the marvel of juice-diet that he began to insist the rest of the members of his family on taking juice-diet.

A few years back, a young man 23 to 24 years old, came to me. He used to get fever at an interval of every ten to twelve days. The temperature sometimes rose to 102-103 degrees and remained so for about three days. Medicines did lower the temperature but did not completely cure the fever. This condition had been going on since two to two and a half years. The continuous taking of poisonous drugs had weakened his body to a large extent.

Following doctors' prescriptions he took different types of medicines and injections, got himself X-rayed and got his blood and sputum (saliva) pathologically examined. But his ailment persisted. One doctor advised him tonsillectomy. This young man followed his advice and went for tonsillectomy. But there was no relief from fever. No one was able to find out the root-cause of the fever.

As the causes of this disease were incomprehensible, I politely refused to take up this case. How can one treat a patient whose disease cannot be diagnosed? But this young patient continued to insist me on giving him treatment.

At last I submitted to his insistence. I advised him to live solely on juice-diet after observing fast for two days. I also instructed him to take enema twice or thrice a day. I prescribed the following regimen to be taken from the third day.

Half a cupful bitter neem-juice on an empty stomach, a glassful of mixed juices (slightly warm) of mosambi and oranges three times a day and hot soup of steamed leafy vegetables twie a day. Along with the prescription, I instructed him to observe water-fast during the relapse of the fever and to switch over back to juice-diet when the temperature became normal.

To his surprise, this time he got fever after about twenty days but it was like the last residue. The temperature rose to 100°F only and that also dropped down to normal the next day. After about six months, when he came to see me, he looked radiant. I asked him how he felt then. He replied that he was much better and added that he no longer suffered from fever. He stated that as his body was very weak and pale, everyone believed as if he was suffering from some terrible disease and that no father was prepared to marry his daughter to him. He then gave me his wedding-card inviting me to attend his marriage. "Now the problem has been solved. Do attend my wedding-ceremony."

4. EPILOGUE

On completion of writing a book, a writer invariably experiences the feeling of joy and contentment of having completed a work. When a writer completes a book, he always asks himself whether he has included all that he had intended to say, whether he has properly emphasised the important points, whether he has presented his view completely and clearly.

The writer of a book has a two-fold duty : (1) Duty to himself – for which the book has been written and (2) Duty to the readers – to write a book aiming at making the lives of the readers more joyful and healthy.

Our humble opinion is that we have fulfilled our duty to ourselves by writing this book. We hope that we have also succeeded in fulfilling our duty to the readers. Despite all our efforts, it is possible that some faults or defects might have crept in the book. We shall try our best to eliminate such mistakes from the next edition of this book, if brought to our notice.

The readers also have a duty – a duty to read the book without prejudice, to examine the element of the book and to inform us about their response and reaction.

It is as clear as daylight that no benefit can be gained by merely reading this book. The book serves no purpose unless the reader puts into practice whatever he has read and comprehended. Planned and regular juice-diet certainly gives expected results. One would not be disappointed if one resorts to juice-diet. There is no reason why one should be deprived of the benefits of this never-failing treatment.

Keep the book handy, read it frequently concentrating on its essential features.

Remember : Maintenance of health is a life-long, sacred duty. It happens that when one reads a book for the first time, he reads it with overenthusiasm. But later on, one forgets everything one has read. This is meaningless.

The purpose of the endeavour of the authors of this book will be served if the reader implements juice-treatment to gain health and maintain it. It will encourage us to make the book better.

_____

INDEX

acidity 156
acne 156
alfalfa 128
amaranth 122
amygdalin 16
anemia 156
aphthae 156
apple 54
arginine 104
ascrobic acid 16
asthma 156
beet 56
bel 58
Berg (Dr) 27
beri-beri 17
Bernarr (Dr) McFadden 127
bezil 123
bioflavonoids 93
biotine 16
Bircher (Dr) Banner 29
bronchitis 156
bitter gourd 59
cabbage 61
calcium 22
cancer 70, 156
Cancer Hospital 115
carbohydrates 13
cardiac troubles 157
carotene 14, 65
carpain 104
carrot 64
Chittenden (Dr) Russell 49
chlorine 24
chlorophyll 120
cholera 157
cholesterol 9, 13
choline 16
cobalt 25
coconut 70
cold 157
colitis 157

constipation 157
contagious diseases 157
copper 25
coriander 121
coughing 157
Crossman (Dr) F. W. 81
Cuboni (Dr) E. 98
cucumber 72
Devaprosad (Dr) Sanyal 58
diabetes 8, 157
diarrhoea 158
dill 130
Dimak (Dr) 59
diphtheria 158
drumstick leaves 129
Dutt (Dr) R. L. 59
eczema 158
Edmund Hillary 95
Ekart (Dr) 27
Elmby (Dr) A. 20
Emblica Mirobelan (amla) 74
enzymes 25
eyes 158
Fanmuller 94
fat 13
Fatzer (Dr) A.S. 19
Fenugreek 126
fever 158
fibrin 104
fig 76
Firenczi (Dr) 56, 57
fluorine 25
folate 18
Folk (Dr) 27
fracture 159
Frederick (Dr) Marwood 10
French beans 78
freshness 158
garlic 79
Garneth (Dr) Cheney 61, 62, 63
George (Dr) B. Schaller 32

George (Dr) J. Druce 11
ginger 82
Giri (Dr) K. V. 74
gout 159
grape cure 88
grapes 84
grapes cure-cancer 86
Hannon (Dr) 63
Hare (Dr) D. C. 51
headache 159
Henry (Dr) Edward Cox 93
Henry (Dr) Sherman 40
Heubner (Dr) 98
Heupe (Dr) W. 51
high blood pressure 159
honey 141
hyper cholesterloaemia 159
hypoglycemia 9
impurity of blood 159
indigestion 160
infertility 160
influenza 160
inositol 16
insomnia 160
internal haemorrhage 160
iodine 24
jambul 91
James (Dr) B. Sumner 25
James (Dr) Litham 34
jaundice 160
Johana (Dr) W. Brandt 86
John Yudkin (Prof.) 8
Joseph (Dr) Evers 52
juice treatment 155
Kanai (Dr) 52
Kellogg (Dr) J. H. 55, 86, 93, 117
kidney-stone 160
Kinderheilh (Dr) J. F. 51
Kirschner (Dr) H. E. 48
Kubler (Dr) W. 65

Kulranjan Mukerji (Dr) 76, 92, 112
Kunstmann (Dr) 57
Kuratsune (Dr) M. 52
lactose 123
laetrile 16, 140
Laetrile (Dr) Calus 140
leafy vegetables 120
lemon 92
liver extract 92
Lust (Dr) J. B. 84, 88
Lytton (Dr) 104
melon 95
menstrual disorders 161
Metchnikoff (Dr) 66
migraine 161
Minchin (Dr) 80
minerals 20
mint (parsley) 125
miracles of carrot-juice 67
Moriondi (Dr) C. 98
multiple sclerosis 52
National Cancer Institute 65
National Heart, Lungs, Blood Institute 65
nausea 161
nervous disorders 161
Newber (Dr) L. H. 47
niacin 17
nicotinamide 17
nicotinic acid 17
Nolfi (Dr) Kristine 52
obesity 161
O'Dell (Dr) 62
onions 97
orange 99
osteoporosis 161
panguamic acid 16
pantothenic acid 16
papain 103, 104
papaya 103
peptic ulcers 161

phosphorus 22
piles 161
pineapple 105
pneumonia 162
pomegranate 107
potassium 23, 35
potatoes 108
pregnancy 162
Price (Dr) G. 59
prostant gland 94, 162
prostate gland troubles 162
protein 13
prothrombin 15
pumpkin 111
pyorrhoea 162
pyridoxine 16, 17
radish 127
radish leaves 127
Rasiklal Parikh (Rajvaidya) 82
Reisser (Dr) 16
rejuvenation 162
rejuvenation by milk 144
renal diseases 162
retinol 14
rheumatism 162
riboflavin 16
Rudat (Dr) 52
saturated fatty acids 13
scurvy 162
Sekla (Dr) 27
Shircore (Dr) 96
skin diseases 163
sodium 24
solanine 93
spinach 124

splenomegaly 163
sulphur 24
sunstroke 163
thalidomide 5
thiamine 17
Thomas (Dr) 131
throat troubles 163
tocokinin 54
Todhunter (Dr) E. M. 19
tomatoes 113
tuberculosis 163
turmeric 115
typhoid 163
Upton Sinclair (Dr) 87
vitamins 14
vitamin A 14, 35
vitamin B 16, 35
vitamin B_1 17
vitamin B_2 17
vitamin B_{12} 18
vitamin C 16
vitamin D 15
vitamin K 15
vitamin P 18
vitamin U 62
Warburg (Dr) E. 20
watermelon 117
weakened sexual drive 163
wheatgrass 130
white gourd 118
Wigmore (Dr) Ann 130
William (Dr) C. Ritz 48
Wilson (Dr) Popenoe 93, 107
worms 164
zinc 25

Published by   Navneet Publications (India) Ltd., Dantali, Gujarat.
Printed by   Navneet Publications (India) Ltd., Dantali, Gujarat.